The TIME TRAVELLER'S HERBAL

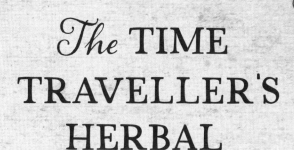

The TIME TRAVELLER'S HERBAL

Stories and recipes from the historical apothecary cabinet

AMANDA EDMISTON

DAVID & CHARLES

www.davidandcharles.com

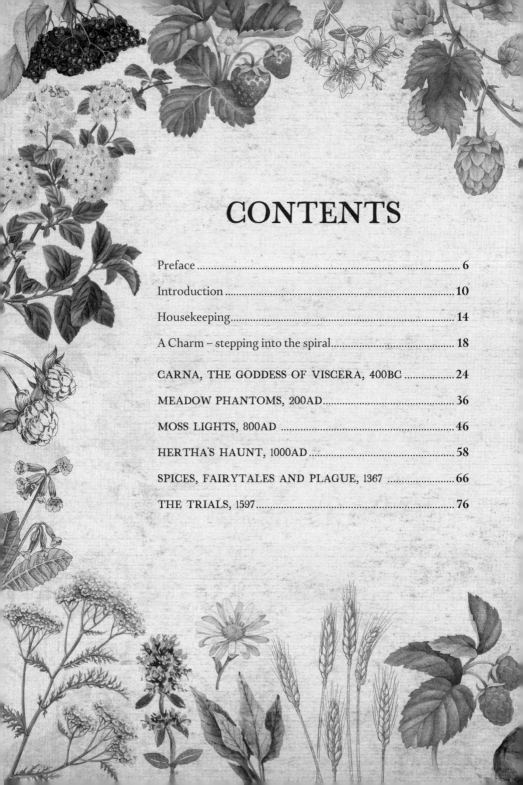

CONTENTS

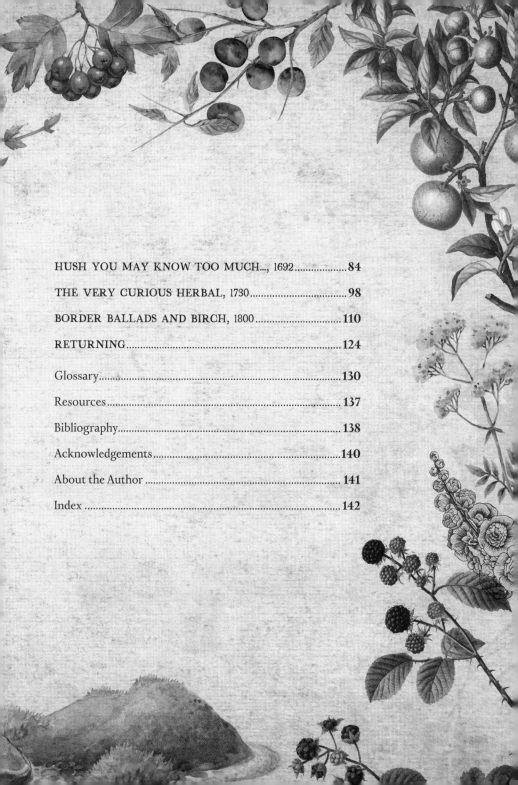

PREFACE

Plants and stories have always been important to me.

I first learnt about plants from my mum and my gran, and my grandad, a sculptor, told me stories whilst he carved in his studio. My mum has been a professional storyteller for over thirty years, but my own journey really began when I found myself a single parent with my eldest child, who was just a few months old at the time. (This was a few years before I met my wonderful partner who officially became her dad.)

I had found a rather magical toddler group that took place in a hidden garden – there were herbs and sculptures – it was a safe place for the children to play. We were a diverse group with families from many different parts of the world. Each week parents took turns to run activities as volunteers and it was here I started my own professional storytelling journey.

Having 'officially' studied herbal medicine before becoming pregnant, I knew I didn't want to go into clinical practice. I wanted somehow to share my excitement about plants and the incredible way they could influence our health, the important roles they played in the fabric of our lives and how they connect us.

I also saw in the folklore that surrounded plants – in the fairy tales that contained them, and the legends and myths from every country in the world surrounding them – that what we now describe in academic or scientific terms was actually held within stories and lore, described in simple terms, or alluded to in metaphor. I knew that the stories we hear even as children stick with us, as we remember both details and nuance. These

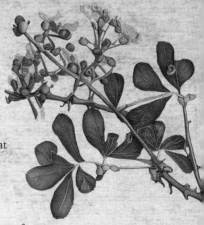

stories build a safe, imaginary world in which to explore and discover new things. Furthermore, I reasoned, even a child will remember that nettles can be woven into fabric, that trees give gifts or that frankincense can help cells renew themselves, if these things are woven into the threads of a story; whereas very few people will endeavour to read hundreds of pages of academic, scientific research.

For example, one of the first stories I told is also one of the most ancient in my repertoire. The origins date back to at least 5000BC. The **Bennu**, a phoenix-like bird, is created by the sun to sing his praises, and in return the sun offers the bird eternal life. For five hundred years the **Bennu** circles the earth singing the praises of the sun. But as people get louder and grow in number, as they build more cities and begin to listen less, the **Bennu** has to raise its voice higher and higher and becomes increasingly weary. Fearing its life is coming to an end, the bird alights on a tree and asks the sun: Why does it feel as if it will die? Where is the eternal life it was promised? The sun looks down on its noble bird and tells it to fly one more time, to gather on its journey aromatic woods to build a nest, and also resin from the frankincense (*Boswellia sacra*) and myrrh (*Commiphora molmol*). It must form the frankincense and myrhh into an egg. The **Bennu** then sings to the sun one last time. The sun shines down on the **Bennu** and its nest and they are burnt down to ash, whereupon the egg opens and the bird is reborn. This cycle is repeated every five hundred years, and is how the **Bennu** has eternal life.

This is an interesting tale from the perspective of how stories relate the use and potential of the medicinal properties of plants, as not only have frankincense and myrrh been used in traditional medicine for their ability to renew cell damage, but recent exacting medical research has also found them to be effective in certain degenerative disorders.

The science really is held within the stories.

My mum started to encourage me to tell stories. She has always inspired me, but now she mentored me, teaching me the art of professional storytelling.

Those first sessions, shared with a friendly group of all ages, from a diverse range of cultures, proved something else: we all know stories, they often travel and have variants in other countries, and we all use plants – the same medicinal properties or culinary uses provide a common ground for people to connect. Plants and stories start conversations, intergenerationally, across cultural and social divides. They bring us together.

The storytelling sessions proved very popular. The multisensory experience of being able to taste and smell the plants in the stories whilst they were told, added layers to the experience, my passion seemed to pique interest. In August 2011 I was invited to travel to London to share stories at the legendary Chelsea Physic Garden for their 'Spice' weekend. When I returned, The Scottish Ballet's education department asked me to make a short film to complement their production of *Sleeping Beauty*.

It seemed that I had knitted my own job!

When people say they've never heard of a herbal storyteller before, I explain how it all started: it was just a selection of things that made me happy and excited, that fitted together and became a thing I loved.

Botanica Fabula was born.

So at the time of writing, Scotland is my home, but I have been creating projects, performances, workshops and bespoke events – in which the participants and I share interactive, multisensory, herbal storytelling pieces often accompanied by visual elements (specially created story boxes or art created by the participants in response to the stories) – for venues and people around the world for over twelve years.

I've collected social history surrounding plant use by researching archives and talking to folk, usually as part of intergenerational projects. I've followed trails of legends and plant-lore, gathered stories and asked questions in gardens and museums. I've been lucky enough to have created work for some wonderful places and met some incredible and fascinating people. And all the while I've been playing with plants and finding ways of sharing their stories.

A lot of the stories I tell take the form of a fairy tale or legend, sometimes traditional, sometimes new but following a traditional form. I then weave in the social histories I've heard, with the research and plantlore. Sometimes I find snippets of folklore and feel there is a lost story there somewhere and 'story-mend' it, embellishing it to keep it alive for new audiences, or tweaking things – as oral storytellers always have – to allow the stories to grow and stay relevant.

The Time Traveller's Herbal is a written reflection of my practice, a combination of all these things. The folklore entwined into the narrative is 'real folklore', carefully researched traditions and spoken word charms associated with places and plants for centuries, and practiced in the eras we will travel through as this book unfolds. The places are real. The social history and time periods have been carefully considered. I just like to set things in a story, because stories are part of our lives.

The stories you will read here are accompanied by recipes you might like to try: ones that relate to the historical period or offer a taste of the plants in the stories – sensory elements that bring the stories to life. There are legends in here too that I've been told since childhood, insights into some of my adventures as a travelling herbal storyteller and a look at the plants and landscapes that I'm familiar with. I hope it makes you want to sit outside, preferably somewhere that you love, and look at the plants around you, wherever you are. Dandelions growing through cracks in paving stones, or towering trees lining railway lines, or parks are as magical as meadows and mountains.

I urge you to experiment with plants: dig out a good identification guide, create small things, read a good basic herbal, learn what can help and what can harm. Make notes, create pictures and stories of your own and add them to these pages, then share your stories, your recipes and pictures with someone else.

Because plants and stories connect us all.

Love

Amanda

X

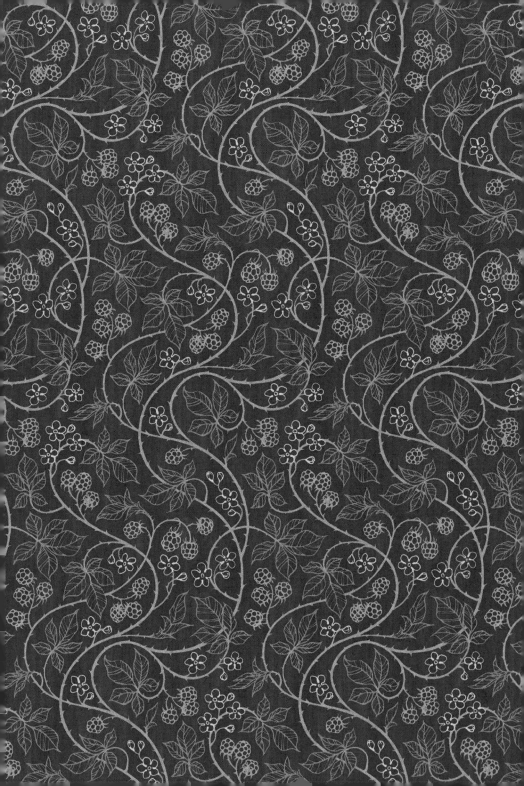

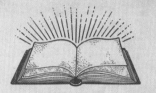

INTRODUCTION

It all started over 40 years ago, with me sitting on the yellow lino-leum floor underneath my gran's kitchen table. The Aberdeen granite chill seeping up from the floor contrasting with the hot draft of confection-scented heat as she opened the oven door to reveal an Autumn-hued gingerbread, ruby crusted with glace cherries at my behest. It perfumed everything with fragile cinnamon-tinged threads of aroma. I vividly remember picking the buttery crystallised crusts of sugar from the thick soft pages of Florence Marian McNeill's *The Scots Kitchen*, too young to understand the words. Gradually, as I learnt to read, I came to recognise that this treasured book not only held reci-pes, but also intriguing hints of folklore and stories. It offered details of collected traditions that promised 'dreaming bread' for newlyweds and **bannocks** to provide Hallowe'en divination – I was captivated.

It was a book my gran had been gifted by her mother-in-law when she had married my grandad during the Second World War. She was a young nurse, a farmer's daughter with Romany roots, and he a sculptor, a minister's son, who had taken on the wartime role of navigator for the RAF. I remember watching my gran write notes in the book's margins about quantities needed, interspersing our culinary moments with trips to the garden to harvest what she needed. We collected fresh handfuls of mint to cut through the butter while she explained that mint helped the digestion, she would then use it to anoint new potatoes. She'd hand me a colander to gather blackcurrants, assuring me I could eat the wild haws that grew alongside them as well as the cultivated berries in the garden. She told me about eating hawthorn leaves on cycle rides to school in her childhood, when there was little else to grace a sandwich, telling me they tasted of bread and cheese. I still love their nutty, heart-healing flavour to this day. When my gran died, her gardening and cookery books were what I reached for.

My mum is a weaver of stories, and I learnt from her too. She expanded and embellished my grandfather's stories, of mermaids and wulvers, castles and ancient stones, as he stood in his studio, giving me clay to mould while he smoked his pipe and carved huge trunks of wood. It's fair to say I've been immersed in such lore since I was barely formed – I've had plants, stories, folklore and food scribed across the soft skin-tissue where my fontanelles once dipped.

As I got older something of the domesticity glimpsed within *The Scots Kitchen's* yellowing leaves left me sensing a **mycelial** connection between the world that Florence Marian McNeill, folklorist and author of *The Silver Bough*, had evoked – tactile, shared on almond- and vanilla-scented lignin and delivered alongside a cup of hedgerow-plucked **tisane** – and a folkloric binding to the 'superstitious keeping of days', unwilling to relinquish its logic to the scientific enquirers, but prescient, nonetheless.

I wanted to slip back through time, to cycle down those May-blossom-clad lanes with my gran, then travel back to McNeill's world at the start of the twentieth century, discovering more stories and recipes, healing potions and enticing lore. I longed to venture further back to find the ancient people my grandad had spoken of, uncover the secrets about plants that they might know, and fly through time gathering words and flavours, secrets and scents... The plants, stories, recipes and enchantment were all interwoven for me.

So I want to lead you now into this world: as I create it on these pages it becomes real. My mum always told me 'a story is true whilst it's being told'. If you taste the plants as we go, look out for them growing between the cracks in the pavement, and infuse the leaves that grow within each story, the world of *Botanica Fabula* will open up and flourish, guiding you on a journey, back into the world of apothecary storytelling, into *The Time Traveller's Herbal*.

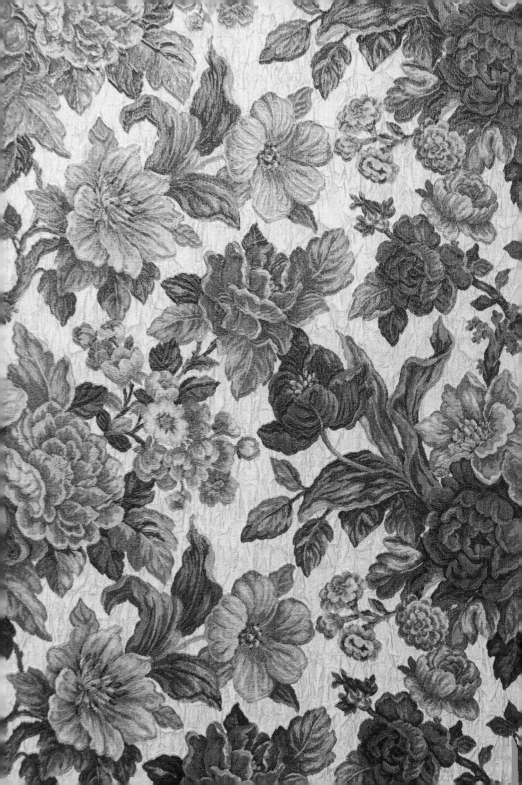

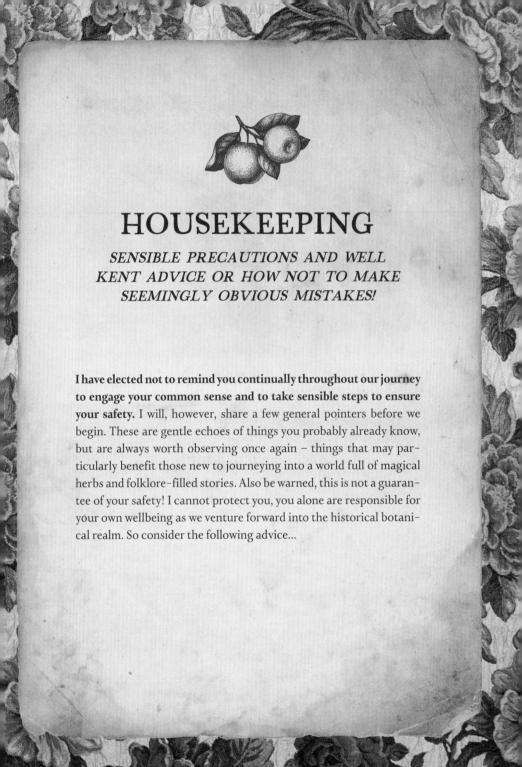

HOUSEKEEPING

SENSIBLE PRECAUTIONS AND WELL KENT ADVICE OR HOW NOT TO MAKE SEEMINGLY OBVIOUS MISTAKES!

I have elected not to remind you continually throughout our journey to engage your common sense and to take sensible steps to ensure your safety. I will, however, share a few general pointers before we begin. These are gentle echoes of things you probably already know, but are always worth observing once again – things that may particularly benefit those new to journeying into a world full of magical herbs and folklore-filled stories. Also be warned, this is not a guarantee of your safety! I cannot protect you, you alone are responsible for your own wellbeing as we venture forward into the historical botanical realm. So consider the following advice…

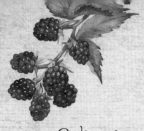

When foraging in the wild

1. Only take leaves, berries and flowers from common plants that grow in abundance. Do not take more than a few from any one place and only take roots from plants growing in your own garden. It may seem that there are 'huge numbers' of certain plants but they can still easily be foraged to extinction.

It is worth remembering as we time travel, that in the early 1800s germander speedwell (Veronica chamaedrys), a plant we now think of as extremely uncommon was popular as a tea. It was so valued for its ability to promote eye health that it was picked into obscurity.

I have tried to focus on simple hedgerow plants that grow in large numbers even in urban environments, or as garden/window box cultivars, in these pages so you can work through the book with an easy conscience. But it is always best to exercise a little self-awareness when foraging for any species, even the humble nettle.

2. Try to forage for plants away from roads with heavy traffic, or areas that may have been previously used by heavy industry, or as dumping sites, as pollution can lead to problematic levels of metals or toxic elements.

3. Where there is livestock or a particularly large number of dog walkers it is best to focus on what I describe as plants 'growing above bottom height'!

4. Gently wash all plant materials before use. I do eat unwashed daisies and hawthorn leaves in the wild, but if you also choose to do so, then that is your decision!

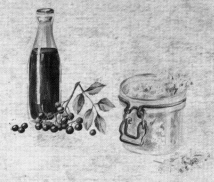

In the kitchen

1. Always sterilise containers and jars before use. A good clean followed by boiling water is sufficient for home use.

2. Glass and stoneware are the best receptacles as they have least effect on their contents. Try to avoid plastic containers as they can leach dysregulating factors into your creations.

3. Use the best ingredients you can afford. Locally sourced, organic produce from small suppliers has far more therapeutic potential than mass-produced goods, and is better for the planet. That said, when budgets are tight, wild food and herbal teas can be an affordable or free way to enhance your life – you don't always need the fancy extras.

4. If you have a good plant guide and a basic reputable guide to simple healing with herbs, then try experimenting with herbal flavours. The basics such as a tea or **tisane** I cover in this book, and these brews can be used as a simple method of taking many safe, non-toxic plants.

5. Do not attempt to treat serious medical conditions yourself. Whilst simple homemade plant remedies can ease the symptoms of a cold, help bring restful sleep and have numerous other health benefits, it takes a proper consultation with a qualified herbalist to safely use a therapeutic dose of plant medicine, with a degree of regularity, for an effective length of time. Herbalists can treat many conditions effectively. However, you should ensure you seek the first-hand help of someone who is properly trained. A good place to start looking for a registered medical herbalist in the UK is the website of the National Institute of Medical Herbalists, or in the USA look for the American Herbalists Guild. Wherever you are in the world it's worth visiting the NIMH website as a highly regarded source for information. See my list of resources at the end of this book for contact details.

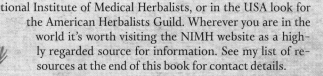

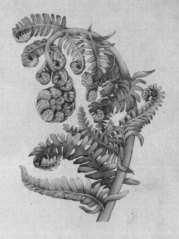

A CHARM

STEPPING INTO THE SPIRAL

When I'm sharing stories and potions in herbal storytelling workshops I often get participants to walk round a spiral laid out on the floor using materials with particular associations to periods of history, maybe recycled silk and nettle twine. We add objects and old postcards, words from the **frith,** lines of poetry, or spoken word charms, plus leaves from plants connected to the stories I'm about to tell. Traversing this spiralling path helps us to visualise passing back through the ages, acting as a physical connection to a journey into the imagination. This makes it more real, the objects and words act as guides, allowing us to immerse ourselves in the story, actively travelling back through time.

I'd love you to join me now as we play a simple game with our imagination.

SO MAYBE YOU CAN FIND...

A sprig of St. John's Wort (*Hypericum perforatum*), chanced upon not sought?

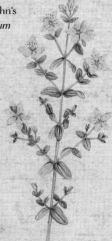

Or a sip of Mugwort (*Artemesia vulgaris*) tea to help you dream and travel without fatigue, in unexpected ways?

'If a footman take a sip of Mugwort then put it into his shoes in the morning, he may goe forty miles before noon and not be weary.'
from The Art of Simpling, *William Coles, 1656*

The axillary plant Colum-Cill,

Unsought for, unwanted,

They will not take you from your sleep,

Nor will you take a fever,

I will put the brown-leaved one,

A plant found beside a cleft,

No man will have it from me

Without more than my blessing.

from The Silver Bough, *F. Marian MacNeill*

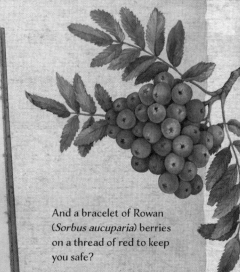

And a bracelet of Rowan (*Sorbus aucuparia*) berries on a thread of red to keep you safe?

'Rowan berries, red thread, tyn the de'il in his stead...'
Scots Traditional

A DAISY DUO

You may also find it useful, ahead of our journey, to equip yourself with my favourite 'bump treatments', a handy herbal first aid kit item for travellers. When I was little my gran would tell me to eat a daisy when I bumped my knee and for years, I assumed this was just a distraction technique. Later I learnt that this was rooted in truth. The humble garden lawn daisy (*Bellis perennis*) is related not just to the soothing chamomiles but also to *Arnica montana*, the go-to remedy for those of us prone to accidents.

DAISY BUMP SYRUP

100g (3½oz) daisy petals (both the yellow and white parts, but discard the green as this can be bitter and spoil the colour of your syrup). Gather before mowing the lawn (as long as chemicals aren't used).

150ml (5fl oz) filtered or spring water.

150g (5¼oz) sugar or six to eight tablespoons of honey (if using honey, a locally produced honey will have added benefits).

Measure 150ml (5fl oz) freshly boiled, filtered water and pour over half the petals. Steep for up to an hour.

Strain water into a pan, squeezing daisies out well, and bring to a gentle boil. Add the remaining petals and simmer softly for 15 minutes.

Strain once more and add sugar or honey. Cook gently until fully dissolved and reduce until preferred consistency.

A squeeze of lemon juice will help preserve it a little longer. It will keep for up to six weeks in the fridge. Take a teaspoon every couple of hours after a bump for the first day, then a teaspoon twice a day until the bruising fades. And remember, if you have a bump on a walk, you can always just eat a daisy! The syrup also has a delicious floral note and can also be used to pour on porridge or pancakes.

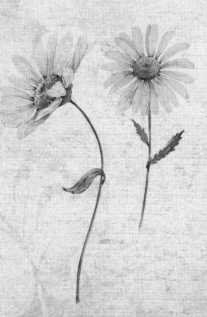

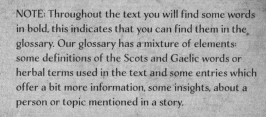

NOTE: Throughout the text you will find some words in bold, this indicates that you can find them in the glossary. Our glossary has a mixture of elements: some definitions of the Scots and Gaelic words or herbal terms used in the text and some entries which offer a bit more information, some insights, about a person or topic mentioned in a story.

DAISY BUMP BALM

A soothing salve to apply topically as soon as you bump a knee!

25g (1oz) daisy-infused oil (sunflower or rapeseed oil work best in my experience). Or use an amount equal to the quantity of wax (see below).

To infuse the oil, gather enough daisies to fill a jar twice, then allow to dry slightly. Fresh or thoroughly dried will work, but even allowing them to wilt well, over 24 hours, reduces the water content sufficiently to make the eventual balm blending process easier.

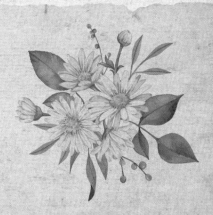

Put the daisies in a glass jar and fill with oil, making sure all the flowers are covered. Place on a sun-drenched window to infuse for two weeks, then strain.

Once you have your infused oil take:

25g (1oz) beeswax, or an amount equal to the quantity of oil.

Melt the oil and beeswax gently over a low heat in a double boiler, or a bowl resting on a small saucepan with a couple of centimeters (an inch) of water in the bottom (do not allow to boil dry!). Stir slowly and once thoroughly combined whisk lightly until it starts to set.

Leave to cool for a minute, then pour into small jars and allow to set.

The balm can last for six months to a year if kept cool, but do not allow it to get too warm as it will start to melt again.

Now you have the beginnings of a herbal first aid kit, we're ready to travel.

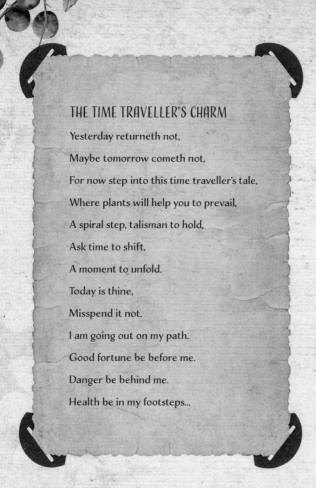

THE TIME TRAVELLER'S CHARM

Yesterday returneth not,

Maybe tomorrow cometh not,

For now step into this time traveller's tale,

Where plants will help you to prevail,

A spiral step, talisman to hold,

Ask time to shift,

A moment to unfold.

Today is thine,

Misspend it not.

I am going out on my path.

Good fortune be before me.

Danger be behind me.

Health be in my footsteps...

I confess I could not find an ancient time-worn Scottish '**eòlas**' or spoken word charm to protect travellers on a rather peculiar journey such as this.

Nor was I prepared to tinker with herbs in order to induce an appropriate twist in the mind to start this story, at least not without you all being present!

I've elected instead to blend my own variant: suggesting protective herbs to safeguard you and drawing patterns gathered from ancient scripts, but I encourage you to discover and create your own. This is not a book of witchcraft, this is a book that will lead you into a world of story. It's a world that has stood the test of time, where we blend narratives and **tisanes**, old, collected, informed and new. And I urge you to develop something of your own – something that organically shifts, allowing you to discover a world of plants, related by stories, for yourself.

We've already spotted a hawthorn (*Crataegus monogyna*) tree or two as I led you in through the introduction, but now I'd like you to keep watch for the faerie tree. This tree, a hawthorn, is said in Irish and Scottish lore to mark the way to the world of the good folk, the fae, a world where time shifts and much can be learnt. Sit beneath its branches, inhale the strange scent of its blossom, start to dream, to imagine unseen worlds and different eras.

Now suitably equipped, I will lead you on a journey, traversing time, to find the hidden stories and folk-lore that reveal the items to be un-covered at the back of the apoth-ecary's almanac... Close your eyes for a moment, sip your **tisane** and travel with me as we go back in time through the centuries to the place where our journey begins: a place where the Roman goddess of vis-cera awaits us!

We slip quickly past the times within living memory, past pina-fore-clad children gathering rose-hips and folk fashioning cold frames to cultivate cucumbers. Onwards, we pass flickering salmon-tailed merfolk whispering of the dangers of destroying meadows. We journey back through eras that are sepia toned with age, with glimpses of pots simmering over flames, smoke filled air, fragrant with pine resin. We speed past wild-eyed women holding out purple toned tomatoes, the spiral twists faster, tumbling into woods where warriors seek knowledge from hazelnut-fed fish.

History and the story begin to merge – we are past the point where certainty is clear. Then familiarity... we see a hawthorn tree – marker of the entrance to the world of the fae, stopper of time – a few of its twigs are held by the woman we seek, we can step out of the spiral and start to listen, watch and learn...

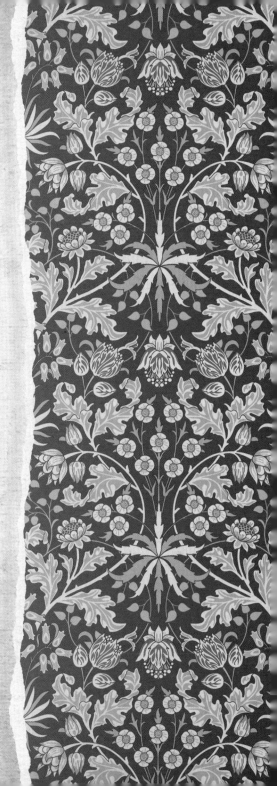

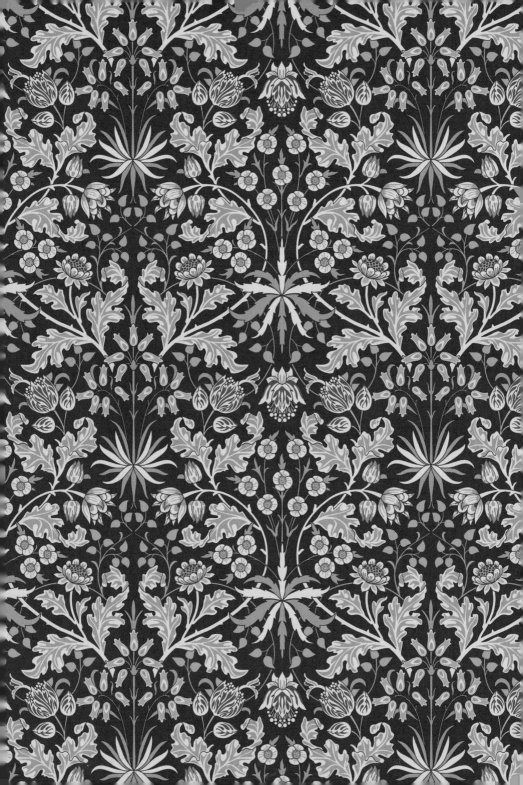

CARNA, THE GODDESS OF VISCERA

400BC

It is June and there is a group walking up a path through shimmering sunshine towards us. We sit under a hawthorn tree on top of the Caelian Hill – one of the seven hills of Rome – next to the temple of Carna. The people approaching are carrying dishes of fava beans and bacon, a dish that when given to the goddess of viscera is said to ensure good digestion for the forthcoming year.

As we try to adjust to the changes in place and time, figuring out that we cannot be seen by the people processing by and realising we will not have to explain our peculiar clothes or sudden arrival, we notice that we can also understand everything that is being said.

A mother carrying a flagon of wine and a plate of food is telling the story of Carna to her children…

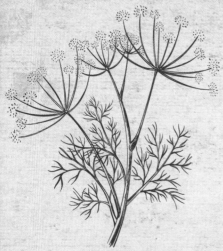

It is said that the goddess was once just a nymph – one acclaimed for her beauty and pursued by young men, who would try to win her affections with gifts and promises. If they weren't easily dissuaded by her disinterest, she would change her tactics and suggest she might reciprocate their affections eventually if they could find their way into her grotto home. Once they reached the cave, however, she easily lost them within seconds, as the cavern system was labyrinthine, a network of tunnels, impossible to navigate by a mere mortal.

Maybe she was strengthened and fortified by fennel seeds (*Foeniculum vulgaris*) reputed to be used by the gladiators to increase strength and endurance, or maybe it was just the diet of bacon and beans, we do not know! But what we do know is that for many years she never tired of this game, utterly disinterested in suitors of any kind.

Then along came the young god, **Janus** – associated with January, beginnings, boundaries and spatial transitions. It would seem from the stories we hear on this hillside that his actions, connected with the boundaries he was said to watch over, were not always entirely honourable. Because when Carna spurned his affections, he persisted and when she tried to lose him in the labyrinth, he took advantage of his dual visage (because Janus had two faces, one looking forward and one behind) and easily found her in the tunnels.

Telling the story the mother shakes her head. Janus' actions were unworthy, but nevertheless all too familiar in tales of ancient deities.

Having behaved so appallingly to Carna, Janus relented and gifted her with divinity. She became a goddess and received the wisdom of hawthorn – the tree that some folk think smells of flesh. It is said she could lure vampiric **Striga** away from their prey.

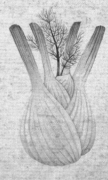

The listening children laugh and shudder, they clearly know the nightmarish habits of these mythical creatures. The mother's voice becomes whispery, dramatic:

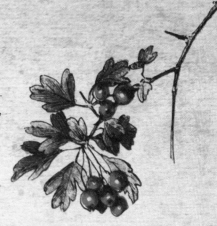

'Because the **Striga** feed on the entrails of sleeping children', she breathes, then adds for effect, 'but only if they misbehave!' And laughs.

The children laugh and run on with the plate of food. All too keen to give their gift to Carna, with the surety that she will lure any Striga away from them, with her bag of hawthorn twigs and a bowl of pig entrails as bait.

The families and visitors disperse, the children begging to be allowed to go down to the grove by the Tiberus where Carna's grotto is said to be. They want to find their way through the labyrinth.

Darkness falls, twinkling lights flicker in the houses below us, people have returned home.

We sit and watch, wondering what will happen next. Will our own labyrinth, the spiral, open and shift once more?

We realise there are shadowy figures lurking beneath the olive trees nearby, watching the windows and listening to parents singing to their children. It is bedtime... a thing that always happens, wherever you are, in whichever time.

The figures move closer.

Out of the temple a woman appears, she starts to move in a spiralling dance of her own.

As we watch, we realise it is Carna laying the hawthorn twigs in an elaborate pattern away from the sleeping children. We see that, sure enough, those strange, unearthly creatures lurking in the shadows are now watching her work.

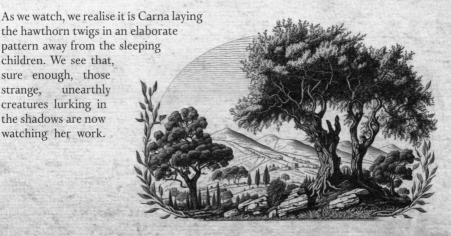

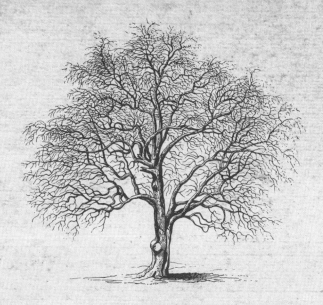

Maybe they are indeed attracted by that infamous death-like scent, caused by the trimethylamine exuded by the late blossoms of the thorn, or maybe like some people they find the scent sweet, an alluring mixture of love and almonds.

One by one they come forward as if compelled. They start to follow the labyrinth of branches, always keeping a safe distance from the goddess. Finally she places down a bowl of pig entrails and retreats back to her temple, and the creatures swarm forward.

As if called by his protective instinct, we see a father appear in a doorway, looking outward to see what has made his children stir. He smooths their hair and steps away again out of sight and bolts the door.

Carna's work is done, the Striga have dispersed.

We follow the pattern of the labyrinth outside the temple a little further and as we do so we realise time is shifting, there are other stories beckoning, dwelling in other places and times. There are plants and environments with remedies to share. I want to take you onward and share the next magical story-world with you, but first I think we may need to start concocting a heart healing, circulation boosting hawthorn infusion, as clearly our journey is full of strange and maybe terrifying things, things that may require heart strength!

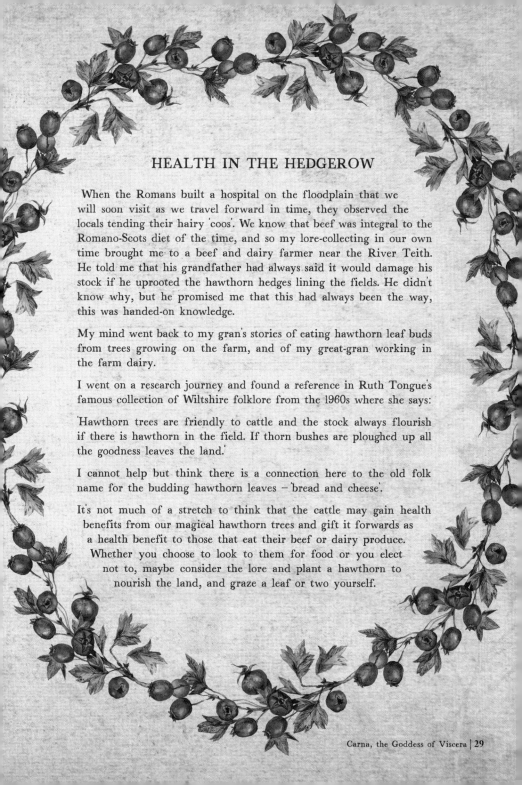

HEALTH IN THE HEDGEROW

When the Romans built a hospital on the floodplain that we will soon visit as we travel forward in time, they observed the locals tending their hairy 'coos'. We know that beef was integral to the Romano-Scots diet of the time, and so my lore-collecting in our own time brought me to a beef and dairy farmer near the River Teith. He told me that his grandfather had always said it would damage his stock if he uprooted the hawthorn hedges lining the fields. He didn't know why, but he promised me that this had always been the way, this was handed-on knowledge.

My mind went back to my gran's stories of eating hawthorn leaf buds from trees growing on the farm, and of my great-gran working in the farm dairy.

I went on a research journey and found a reference in Ruth Tongue's famous collection of Wiltshire folklore from the 1960s where she says:

'Hawthorn trees are friendly to cattle and the stock always flourish if there is hawthorn in the field. If thorn bushes are ploughed up all the goodness leaves the land.'

I cannot help but think there is a connection here to the old folk name for the budding hawthorn leaves – 'bread and cheese'.

It's not much of a stretch to think that the cattle may gain health benefits from our magical hawthorn trees and gift it forwards as a health benefit to those that eat their beef or dairy produce. Whether you choose to look to them for food or you elect not to, maybe consider the lore and plant a hawthorn to nourish the land, and graze a leaf or two yourself.

I was always told that May haw brandy should be saved and drunk in small amounts every evening over the twelve days of Christmas, to warm the hearts of those who may be grieving the absence of those not there to share the festivities. Literally hawthorn to mend a broken heart.

My gran always told me that hawthorn could mend a broken heart. But I now know that this is not just poetic, hawthorn can have beneficial effects generally on the heart and circulatory systems, and help balance blood pressure – all rather useful over the festive season.

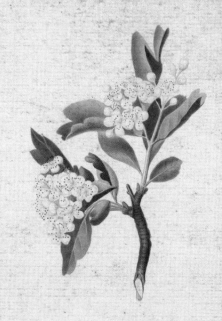

INFUSED BERRIES

Once the berries have been used to infuse the brandy, they can be either returned to the ground or used in a hedgerow jelly (see below), combined with brambles, crab apples, rosehips, elderberries, sloes and maybe a few rowan berries.

MAY HAW BRANDY

Traditionally flowering for May Day, the first of May, hawthorn will actually bloom, depending on where you are in the northern hemisphere, at anytime from late April until the end of May as a general rule. The association with May Day itself might be due to the date shifts created by the introduction of the **Gregorian calendar** in 1752.

If the opportunity, however, does arise to gather your hawthorn flowers on May Day that would be perfect as tradition- ally it was seen as unlucky to bring the blossoms into the house on any other day - to do so would mean someone would become ill, the blossoms perhaps even foretelling death. Maybe those **Striga** are being lured into the house!

Maybe we should prepare our blossoms outside just to be safe. After all, even a small harvest of flowers for this recipe should be done on a bright, dry, sunny morning, to allow the flowers to be at their best.

Gather enough May blooms to loosely fill a glass or stoneware jar with a firmly fitting lid. Shake well to remove any un- wittingly gathered beasties! Then add the blossoms to your jar and fill with brandy.

Leave to infuse for around three weeks. Turn or gently shake daily, and ensure that the flowers remain covered.

At the end of the period, strain the flowers off and return them to the ground - scattering them under the hawthorn tree seems like a poetic thank you! (Or see the note about infused berries.)

Now safely label your infused brandy and store it away, as we will return to it in a few months' time.

As the berries ripen on the tree at the end of summer, get your brandy back out of the cupboard.

Pick a warm, dry morning, when the berries have reached a deep red and will slightly compress when squeezed. Gather enough to half fill the original jar. Lightly wash them, remove all stems and add to another jar (this should be one at least the same size or slightly bigger than you used for the flowers).

Add a tablespoon of brown sugar.

Pour the original flower-infused brandy over the berries and allow to infuse for around four weeks. Remember to turn daily and keep the berries covered.

At the end of four weeks strain and bottle the brandy.

HEDGEROW JELLY

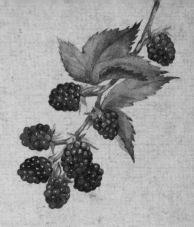

500g (1lb) crab apples or cooking apples

500g (1lb) hedgerow berries (this can be a mixture of elderberries, sloes, haws, rowan, rosehips and brambles)

500g (1lb) granulated sugar (approx)

570ml (1pt) filtered water

Rinse the apples and chop them roughly (no need to peel or core).

Place the apples and berries in a large saucepan with water, ensuring the fruit is covered. Bring the pan to the boil, then simmer until all of the fruit starts to disintegrate when gently mashed with a wooden spoon.

Lightly mash and remove from the heat.

Strain the fruit though a jelly bag or muslin-lined sieve set over a large bowl – press down with a small plate to help push the juice through.

Leave to drip overnight.

Measure the resulting juice – as a guide you are going to need 500g (1lb) of sugar to every pint of liquid.

Return the juice to a saucepan and heat to simmer, then gradually add the sugar, stirring until dissolved.

Increase the heat and bring to a rolling boil for around ten minutes or until the setting point is reached. We always used to do this by dropping half a teaspoonful onto a cold saucer – if it started to set it was ready. Remove the pan from the heat.

Leave the jelly to rest for a few minutes, then pour into sterilised jars and seal well.

Store in a cool, dark place for up to one year.

Keep in the fridge once opened and use it within four months.

The story went in my house that hedgerow jelly eaten every morning on a bowl of porridge would keep winter colds and viruses at bay, certainly the berries are all rich in vitamin C and have anti-viral properties.

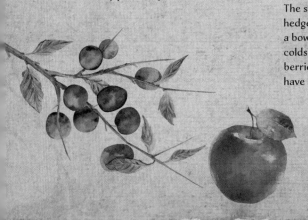

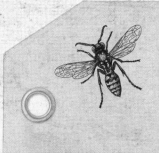

When we used the saucer trick to check the setting point of the jelly, the saucer was afterwards set on the outside windowsill for the wasps - wasps are vital pollinators and we are sharing their fruit, so it's nice to thank them - the jelly leading the wasps away like hawthorn led away the **Striga**!

Also remember:

The fair maid who, the first of May,
Goes to the fields at break of day
And washes in dew from the hawthorn tree,
Will ever after handsome be.

(traditional... and worth a try!)

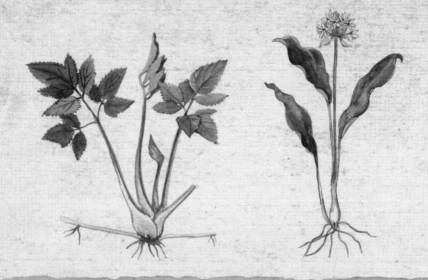

CALEDONIAN HERBAL OIL

New hawthorn leaves just out of bud have a delicious sweet nutty flavour and make a good addition to a spring pesto. This is a budget-friendly, foraged alternative to the Mediterranean pine kernel (*Pinus pinea*), which is currently suffering a decline but which would have been a familiar food to our Roman friends.

Add a handful, along with a similar amount of wild garlic flowers and leaves, some fresh nettle tips and very young tips of ground elder (*Aegopodium podagraria*) – another Roman food staple - to a good glug of extra virgin olive oil. Season with little salt and grind or blend to achieve the desired texture.

This herbal oil is delicious as a vitamin-rich dressing for salad, potatoes or pasta, but it's best used straightaway so just make small amounts!

CAUTION: Ground elder, like nettle, is a mild diuretic and was once used to alleviate gout. It should only be used when just emerging in the Spring as later in the season it can have a laxative effect!

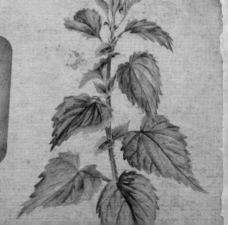

As we take our next step forward in time, we hear whispers of ancient Roman doctors yet to come, of hospitals where women and men study medicine as equals, of people trained in the use of Mediterranean herbs travelling with the invading forces of the Empire and leaving their knowledge and plants behind. We hear a whisper from a healer named Octavia as she bakes barley, honey, vinegar and salt to pulverise with charcoal and flowers to soothe a toothache. We watch as a certain Syrian doctor called Luke, gathers armfuls of sweet, scented lavender to create dream filled sleep pillows for fretful infants...

We cannot stay though, the spiral has caught us, and we are moving forward through time.

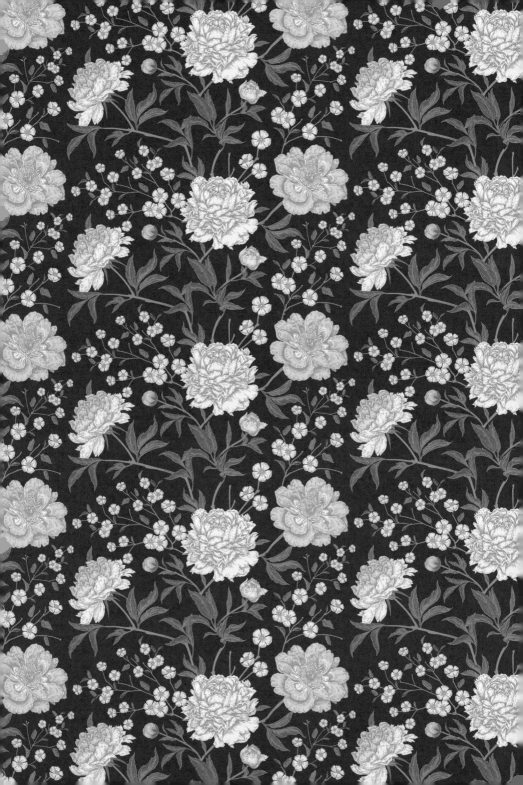

MEADOW PHANTOMS

200AD

Many of my stories, and the recipes and tastes that accompany them, originate in the places I walk. I sit and look around me, notice the plants and the changes afforded by time. I think about the history of the place, the transformations that have occurred over time and the folklore associated with the plants that grow there. It is easy to be drawn into history if you sit and think, feeling the ground beneath your feet, looking at the unchanging elements, the river, the geography.

One of the places I frequent most is a wild floodplain meadow behind a castle where two rivers meet near to my home in Scotland. This fascinating and ecologically important place regularly ventures into my stories. I often imagine inviting a small group of friendly folk to travel back into this meadow's past with me and explore the plants it nurtures and the stories it tells... so I invite you to travel into it with me now as we pass through our next swathe of time.

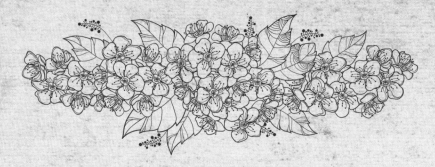

The places we are passing through are barely recognisable without their architectural constructs – the castle and paths that are familiar features in our own time. The tree line is present but is now sculpted differently, however, some things are very familiar: the arc and curve of the rivers and the contours of the hills and mountains. There may be slight changes but their journey follows a different pace to ours and so they seem like a constant, assuring us of geographical certainty, a sense of place.

We find ourselves on the rocky outcrop above the meeting of the two rivers, a confluence marking out the meadow. Behind us is the shadow where the castle will stand. On the opposite bank is a bustling **Pictish** village, with a flower-strewn meadow between.

Before we reach the meadow the scent of **salicylates** beckons. It has a faintly medicinal allure, part sweet notes, partially antiseptic.

I go on, and as I reach the first dip down towards the river, the creamy clouds seem to be blurring the view of the bank, as if some ethereal queen was hiding behind them, not wanting anyone to catch her in her natural form.

I step closer, brushing past the blooms, scattering petals as I seek to catch the being I thought I'd seen... but there's nothing there. The river ripples with the tremble of something silvery slipping away downstream. Eyes may be watching from the nearby wood and there is a young bullock grazing the clover on the other side of the water, but there is no shimmering regal figure.

My imagination has clearly been seduced by the Queen of the Meadows, I've been flower-led into fantasising phantoms sitting on the shore... or maybe I'm running a temperature?

I check myself for fever, then add a few heads of the meadowsweet (*Filipendula ulmaria*) to the flask of hot water I carry whenever I remember.

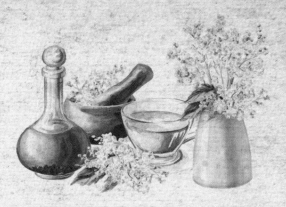

As I sip, the memory of a story whispers in my ear, the penny drops. I am in the presence of **the Morrigan**, phantom queen, capable of transformation, shapeshifter, one of the ethereal and rarely acknowledged, feminine figures in Celtic mythology.

The story goes that the great warrior **Cu Chulainn** was sent to the Isle of Skye to learn the art of combat from the warrior maid, Sgathaich, as in those days it is said that only a man could teach a woman to fight and only a woman could teach a man. He became enamoured with her daughter, Uathach, and the pair were betrothed.

But his life was violent, he was a man of temper and as a warrior he was frequently off on battles. His heroic journeys,

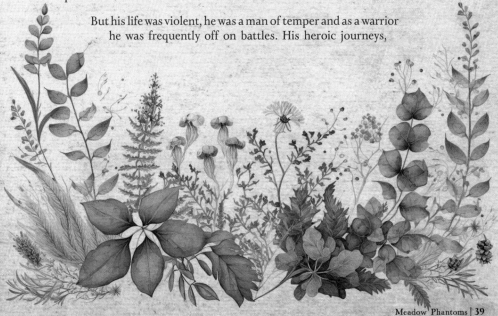

we sense, are littered with dubious encounters with women and I'm not sure his behaviour was admirable. Certainly the story I was told many years ago suggested he was not an innocent party when he encountered the mighty Morrigan, phantom queen. During a battle at a ford – in the form of a beautiful young woman – she offered to help him in the fight if he gave her his love.

When he rebuffed her, claiming his heart belonged to Uathach, she transformed into an eel and tried to twist round his ankles as he crossed the water. But he reached down and wrenched her off, injuring her as he did so. But she was not to be so easily defeated, taking the form of a huge grey wolf, she terrified a herd of cattle and caused them to stampede at the warrior. Taking his slingshot, he hit her hard, wounding her badly in the leg. Finally, she became a white heifer running at the front of the stampede, right towards **Cu Chulainn**, but taking a spear he injured her one last time and she vanished, haar-like into the river.

As the battle drew to an end, Cu Chullainn, weary, cut and bruised, made his way along the riverbank. Eventually he encountered an old woman milking a deer, her body marked with familiar injuries, those he had inflicted on the eel, the wolf and the heifer.

Sore and thirsty, he stopped and asked her for a drink, then blessed her when she gave him a cup and with each cup she gave him, he blessed her again. With each blessing her injuries healed, and as the words left his lips for the third time he realised who she was.

The Morrigan gave him meadowsweet as a gift and although some say he regretted healing her, we can be sure that he carries it on his belt from that day forth. He relies on it, as she has taught him, to bathe in; a handful of fresh blossoms, or a palmful of dried flower heads encased in a muslin bag, added to a bath, to heal his wounds, reduce his fevers and cool him when his temper flares.

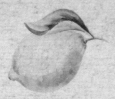

A CORDIAL FOR A PHANTOM QUEEN TO EASE TEMPERS, FEVERS AND HEARTBURN

Thirty heads of meadowsweet blossoms in full flower

Juice of one unwaxed freshly squeezed lemon and a little grated rind

300g (10½oz) blossom honey (locally produced honey has additional benefits)

1 litre (35fl oz) filtered water

Bring the water to the boil and then dissolve half the honey in it. When the honey has dispersed add the meadowsweet, lemon juice and rind, and allow to simmer for a further three minutes.

Remove from the heat and rest overnight (or at least for an hour or two), to allow the meadowsweet to infuse.

Strain and then add the rest of the honey. Return to the boil, allowing the infusion to simmer for a further five minutes or so to reduce.

The mixture should take on the consistency of a cordial. More honey can be added as desired.

Bottle in sterile glass jars or Kilner-style bottles. The cordial lasts for up to three months if kept cool.

Mix with still or sparkling water, or maybe a sparkling wine, and feel the heat dissipate...

We know we are not here for long, for this is a shadow of a place, an ancient time glimpsed as we travel, spiralling to a place where we can stop for a moment. Giving a nod to the last of the mist as it dissipates and the sun lifts a little higher in the early morning sky, we gather an armful of meadowsweet and carry it with us to later steep it in water, add honey and turn it into a cordial, fit for a queen.

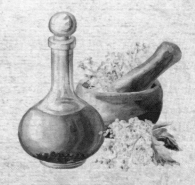

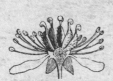
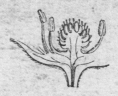
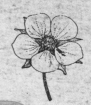

SOOTHING BATH

Meadowsweet blossoms can be added to a bath as the water runs, in a muslin (or similar) bag, to help reduce fevers. Oats can also be added to help soothe irritated or inflamed skin.

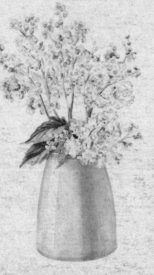

A GLIMPSE OF THE FUTURE?

Still a herbal tonic for heroes, in her collection of early twentieth century wisdom, author Doris E. Coates wrote that meadowsweet 'makes old men young and young men strong'.

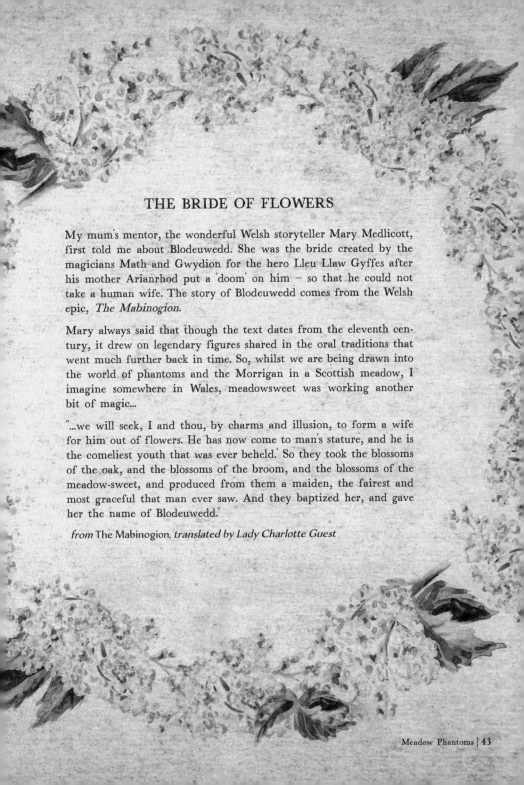

THE BRIDE OF FLOWERS

My mum's mentor, the wonderful Welsh storyteller Mary Medlicott, first told me about Blodeuwedd. She was the bride created by the magicians Math and Gwydion for the hero Lleu Llaw Gyffes after his mother Arianrhod put a 'doom' on him – so that he could not take a human wife. The story of Blodeuwedd comes from the Welsh epic, *The Mabinogion*.

Mary always said that though the text dates from the eleventh century, it drew on legendary figures shared in the oral traditions that went much further back in time. So, whilst we are being drawn into the world of phantoms and the Morrigan in a Scottish meadow, I imagine somewhere in Wales, meadowsweet was working another bit of magic...

"...we will seek, I and thou, by charms and illusion, to form a wife for him out of flowers. He has now come to man's stature, and he is the comeliest youth that was ever beheld.' So they took the blossoms of the oak, and the blossoms of the broom, and the blossoms of the meadow-sweet, and produced from them a maiden, the fairest and most graceful that man ever saw. And they baptized her, and gave her the name of Blodeuwedd.'

from The Mabinogion, *translated by Lady Charlotte Guest*

We think for a moment on these creamy stems from the flower, also called *'Crios Chu-Chulainn'* (Chu-Chulainn's belt) in Gaelic, and once referred to as 'bride-wort' for its popularity as a floral confetti for weddings, and we start to imagine recipes that we can use as the legendary hero once did: a **tisane** or an addition for a soothing bath perhaps? Our cordial is another remedy to add to our apothecary's cabinet, before we embark on the next journey that beckons us forward. Because now we sense that twist in time, the feeling of being pulled again into a tide of years, ebbing and flowing. The shift is visceral...

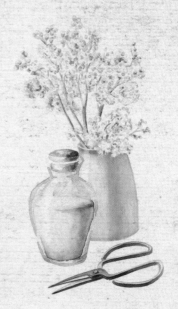

As with many of the plants I mention, meadowsweet can be put into a cup and steeped in freshly boiled water for three or four minutes to create a herbal **tisane**. Meadowsweet is a valuable remedy, having mildly pain-relieving properties and is really good at soothing indigestion!

The landscape is changing, we sense that we have travelled northwards. The sky is brighter, but the temperature has dropped. The ground beneath our feet has changed perceptibly in texture and has a spongy quality. As the spiral twist forward in time, we get the sense that our feet are sinking slightly, we look down to see dark, mineral rich water pool around the soles of our shoes. The urge to move, to seek safety is instinctive and we start to carefully walk forwards...

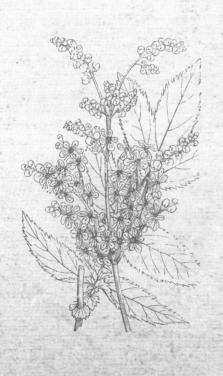

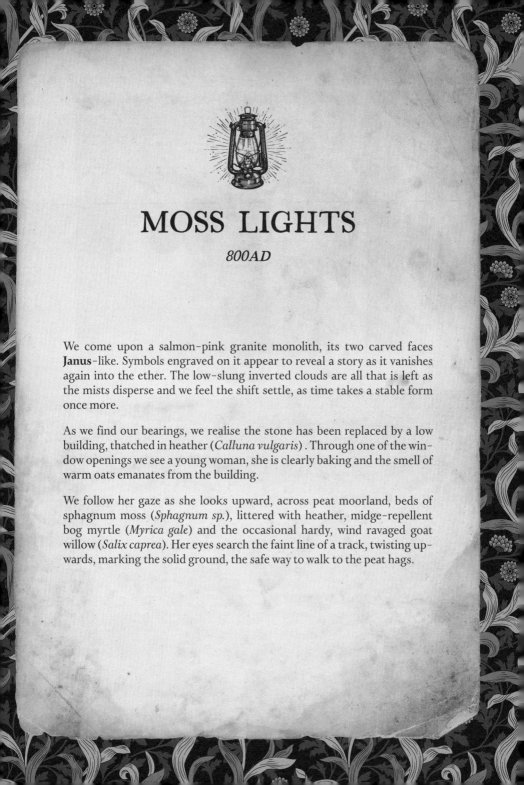

MOSS LIGHTS

800AD

We come upon a salmon-pink granite monolith, its two carved faces **Janus**-like. Symbols engraved on it appear to reveal a story as it vanishes again into the ether. The low-slung inverted clouds are all that is left as the mists disperse and we feel the shift settle, as time takes a stable form once more.

As we find our bearings, we realise the stone has been replaced by a low building, thatched in heather (*Calluna vulgaris*) . Through one of the window openings we see a young woman, she is clearly baking and the smell of warm oats emanates from the building.

We follow her gaze as she looks upward, across peat moorland, beds of sphagnum moss (*Sphagnum sp.*), littered with heather, midge-repellent bog myrtle (*Myrica gale*) and the occasional hardy, wind ravaged goat willow (*Salix caprea*). Her eyes search the faint line of a track, twisting upwards, marking the solid ground, the safe way to walk to the peat hags.

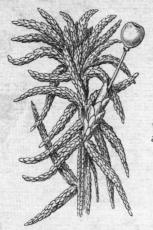

Her family trudge this path daily from March until May, carrying **tairsgears** for cutting and creel baskets for carrying the peat back to dry out in the cottage. Only taking enough to keep the family warm over the winter months and to cook a meal. And to distill an amber drop of the whisky they keep for high days and holidays. They use it to extract the essence of healing herbs, clean wounds and to toast the turning points that need such libations. Because they know, as the family has always known, how important the slow-forming peat is.

The peat is said to be so deep that four men could stand on one another's shoulders and still be lost into its form. The stories say it has been there since the beginning of time, only getting a thumb's length deeper every three hundred years.

The peat contains hidden things, hidden qualities. It is said it holds the world together. That beings live there to protect it – will o' the wisps, bog lights who compel you to stray off the path, moss maidens who could bring plague or offer cures depending on your temperament.

The girl in the cottage keeps watching.

She watches for her family, hoping they will return safely before dusk. She has gazed in this way for more than a year now, since the misty late February night when her grandfather had gone to gather the peat too early in the year and had spotted a light. Thinking it to be a candle flickering, he felt himself compelled to follow it off the path, fatally stepping away from safety and into the bog. Once there he must have lost his footing – or the legendary will o' the wisp really did take him down to the underworld – because the next morning, when the search had finally found the place he had vanished, there was only his hat and an impression on the surface of the bog to indicate where he had been.

Now the lassie watched, hoping and praying that no ill-fated change in the weather would hinder the rest of her family from getting safely home.

We watch as she comes out of the door and gathers club moss (*Lycopodiales sp.*) from beside the stone wall, muttering the words of the club moss charm as she does so:

GARBHAG an t-sleibh air mo shiubhal,

The club-moss is on my person,

Chan eirich domh beud no pud-har;

No harm nor mishap can me befall;

Cha mharbh garmaisg, cha dearg iubhar mi...

No sprite shall slay me, no arrow shall wound me...

But she pauses before she reaches the last line. Something new has arrived on the horizon. Something unexpected in the daily, visual ritual of life...

She stands watching as a stranger approaches, never getting to the final line:

Cha riab grianuisg no glaislig uidhir mi.

No fay nor dun water-nymph shall tear me.

from Carmina Gadelica

The visitor smiles. Not only is this a new face in a place where new faces are few and far between, but it is an undeniably handsome face, with twinkling eyes and a slightly quirky smile. He explains he's had a long journey and wonders if she could get him a cup of water.

Intrigued and hoping to hear a new tale from this traveller, she steps back inside and gets him some water. The pair start to chat and he rests on the bench outside the cottage, accepting a fresh oat **bannock** and making the young woman laugh as he regales her with anecdotes and observations about his adventures.

The sun sinks a little lower in the sky, the young woman ponders internally as to whether this handsome stranger fits the description of the man she saw in her dreams after eating a Bannoch Sallain the Hallowe'en before, for this was a bake her granny had always promised her would bring prophetic dreams.

As they look at the heather around the cottage, the young woman tells the stranger the story her grandmother had told her. Of how the purple flowers of the heather were transformed to white by a young woman's tears after she learnt of her lover's death in battle. How, as her tears had fallen, she had gifted heather with the ability to bring good luck to those who would carry it, good luck so that they would never have the sorrow she herself felt.

As she tells the story we see the stranger's demeanour change, he becomes more attentive. He has clearly become interested in her, with ease he becomes flattering and charming.

The afternoon soon flies by... but as intrigued as she now is, she is still somewhat taken aback when instead of standing up to leave, he drops to one knee and asks her to marry him!

We watch aghast as she seems to be pondering his proposal, her eyes search the horizon, rain clouds smear the view of the high peat hag. She turns to him, and we can almost see her thought process as he begs her to be his bride and offers her anything if she'll just say yes.

She thinks on for another moment, with her eyes on the encroaching clouds. Finally, she says she will marry him, but only if he builds her a road, a safe path from the peat hag to the cottage, so her family can always get back at the end of the day.

We admire her common sense. In this wind-scarred landscape, centuries before the everyday luxuries of our time, this road will be a safety net, allowing the things needed for survival to be safely obtained. Surely, we think the task will take the stranger a year, maybe more to build. They can get to know each other, maybe they will fall in love, maybe we're watching the beginnings of a long happy life, foreseen in a bite of a Hallowe'en bannock.

The stranger gets up, smiles and walks straight up the high hag, clearly making a start on his task. Curious we keep watching – he has no tools, no materials, no place to stay or shelter on this moor. The woman laughs and walks back into the cottage, she has chores to get done, but she always returns to the window, still watching for her family.

An hour passes, she steps outside again, it is nearly time for her family's return. As she looks upward again her eye is caught by something twinkling in the lowering sun. A silvery grey line is curving snake-like down from the peat hag. Moving faster and faster, it gets wider and straighter. Then that twinkle again... With a shiver coursing down her spine she realises the figure at the head of the silver path is the handsome stranger.

The twinkle? The late afternoon sun catching the sparkle of his obsidian hooves. This is no mortal man; she has made a promise to marry the devil himself.

Realising his arrival is imminent she rushes to the cottage, gathering up her treasured mirror and comb. She glances towards the coat of moss she has kept since her childhood, a gift from her grandmother, a woman said to have travelled from the west country and married the girl's grandfather many years before: the story of a Mossy Coat you may be able to catch a note of as you listen to the layers of history surrounding us. She had thought she would keep it and wear it on her wedding day, but now thinks to put the coat on as a protective gift, handed down her maternal line. But before she can shrug it over her shoulders, she senses the presence of the devil at the door. She tries to run, screaming 'I will never marry you...!' but he stands in front of her, a menacing smile on his lips as she tries to put on the coat and get away. Catching her he puts his hand on her shoulder, his voice reverberating around the room:

'If you won't marry me, then you won't marry anyone!'

And with that he turns her to stone.

There she stands, a pink granite monolith, her mirror and her comb like carved adornments on her side.

The air shivers around us, looking like heat waves on a summer's day. The cottage has gone, but the stone still stands. The coat of moss has melded with the earth, still waiting to be draped over the young woman's shoulders, but for now protecting just her feet. A chapel has been built nearby and as we start to feel ourselves spiral forward once more through time, we hear a father recount the tale of the Maiden Stone to his daughter, adding 'the legend says there's a cure for her somewhere in the moss, something that will return her to her human form, if only we can find it...'.

We hear his words and fundamentally understand, for moss we reason, like the meadow, holds many remedies, some known, some forgotten, some yet to be found. There are cures we may all need there, if we just let it grow and keep on looking.

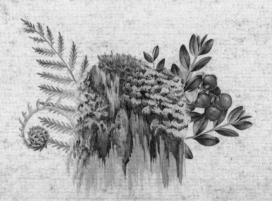

Bannoch Sallain

According to Scottish folk traditions Hallowe'en was celebrated on the night of the dark moon nearest to the end of October, a night when prophecies could be dreamt and our ancestors feasted. A night to try *bannoch sallain*, said to give those that ate it prophetic dreams. Oats bring deep sleep, salt reveals the future.

This traditional **bannock** is recorded by Florence Marian McNeill in *The Scots Kitchen* as being eaten at **Samhain** in the Highlands as a divining charm. It may well owe its powers to the combination of oats, which being high in potassium, magnesium, calcium and melatonin will increase relaxation, release serotonin and help bring sleep, and the kidney-achingly high level of salt (this is not a snack for anyone with high blood pressure!). The ample quantity of salt, which along with the instruction not to drink water following consumption, will lead to mild dehydration that can induce wild dreams!

However, whilst I can explain the chemistry of this charm I cannot promise the accuracy of the resulting dreamt prophecies. For that element you'll just have to trust the magic!

SAMHAIN BANNOCKS

But if you want to give the bannocks a try the recipe and method is thus:

25g (1oz) salt

110g (4oz) oatmeal

1 tsp butter

Drop the ingredients into 140ml (¼ pint) boiling water.

Knead the warm mixture until a dough forms, then bake on a medium heat until golden.

Eat one bannock before turning in for the night, do not drink water or eat anything else after consuming.

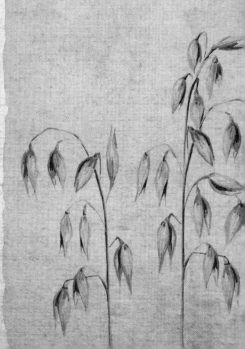

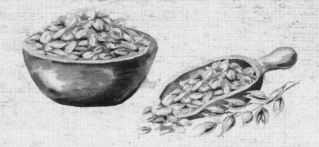

I decided to try the *bannoch sallain* myself one year, taking the ancient family mixing bowl out and stirring the ingredients together. I felt the dough soften to cohesion, moulding it between my hands. The sensation took me back to my grandmother's kitchen in Aberdeen once more, just for a fleeting moment, and I remembered the smell of crisp oatcakes fresh from the oven, begging for butter. As I started to flatten the dough out and cut it into triangles, I suddenly heard her whisper not to eat the scraps that fray along the edges and turned to find myself alone in the kitchen. She has been gone nearly twenty years. The voice must have been a note of birdsong through the open window...

It is said that for the **Samhain bannock** to take effect, no food or drink should pass your lips after its consumption, even a sip of water will hinder the arrival of dreams, nor should any word be spoken. But I realised that just clasping the dough between my palms engendered a glimpse through fluid walls of time, skin soft, to memories.

I baked the bannocks to golden crispness and ate one before it had cooled, packing the rest up to share as I tell Hallowe'en tales to a grown-up audience later on that evening, assured that a little hint of traditional dream divination is magically held within their crumbs.

Colour Changing Warming Heather Tonic

Heather is reputed to have antiseptic and sedative properties. It was once used extensively to treat rheumatism, gout and arthritis, all ailments worsened by cold, wet days spent working on desolate moors.

Rosebay willowherb (*Chamaenerion angustifolium*), whilst not a moorland plant, is easily found on any patch of wild ground, and makes a lovely poetic addition to this recipe. Its use will make the infusion change colour, like heather does in its legend, a change that also mirrors the transformation of the young woman in the story into stone. As a common self-seeding plant, using it is a little more sustainable and accessible in Scotland rather than reaching for the more exotic 'colour changing' plants that are often sought online.

Traditionally used as a 'tea plant', rosebay willowherb has a light flavour and gentle action and was once used to treat childhood tummy troubles.

HEATHER TONIC

Take two tablespoons of purple flowering green tips of heather and simmer in a pan with a pint of water for ten minutes.

Take off the heat and immediately pour over a generous handful of pink rosebay willowherb flowers. Allow to infuse in a cafetière or similar for three minutes.

Strain, then stir in two teaspoons of heather honey.

Now squeeze in the juice of half a lemon and watch your infusion turn a vibrant pink!

A dram of whisky could be added for extra warmth, and is best sipped in front of a fire, maybe with your feet resting in a foot bath of warm water infused with more heather, as traditionally this was a way of warding off chilblains and improving the circulation.

As cures go, this might not turn you back to mortal from stone, but it will help you feel a more human temperature on a cold dark evening!

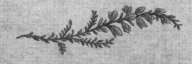

MOSS MOVES IN
MYSTERIOUS WAYS

Vital, carbon-storing peat hags are made up almost entirely of ancient layers of sphagnum moss (*Sphagnum sp.*), which has a long tradition of use as a wound dressing, and to line babies nappies – an ancient purpose that has had more recent applications (but more of that if you choose to travel with me beyond the pages this book!). Everyone should also know about glacier moss balls (*Racometrium sp.*). These incredible natives of an intimidating landscape have been recently found to move on average 2.5 centimeters (about an inch) a day in a 'herd-like fashion'. Moss is mysterious indeed!

The future of our maiden-stone may therefore, given the nature of these incredible plants, depend upon the moss revealing its secrets, as my grandfather always suggested.

In another of Scotland's ancient landscapes, Flanders Moss – the vast expanse of **carse** in rural Stirlingshire – I met a man who owned an 85-year-old herbarium. He showed me the sphagnum held within its pages. It was still alive, despite being captured within a book, kept alive with an occasional spray of water.

Science upholds this anecdotal evidence as Antarctic research in 2017 found 1500-year-old frozen moss that could be brought back to life.

Moss may indeed hold a hope for the future.

Divination techniques work their way through so many of our stories. Tales are told of folk stealing kale stalks from the neighbour's garden to read the ilk of their future partners. Certain actions and behaviours could foretell futures... but I think all we need to do is wait, because our future will be revealed as the next stage of our journey unfolds...

On a final note, before we begin to travel forward again in time, beware of flattering handsome strangers who offer the impossible, they are quite often not what they seem to be!

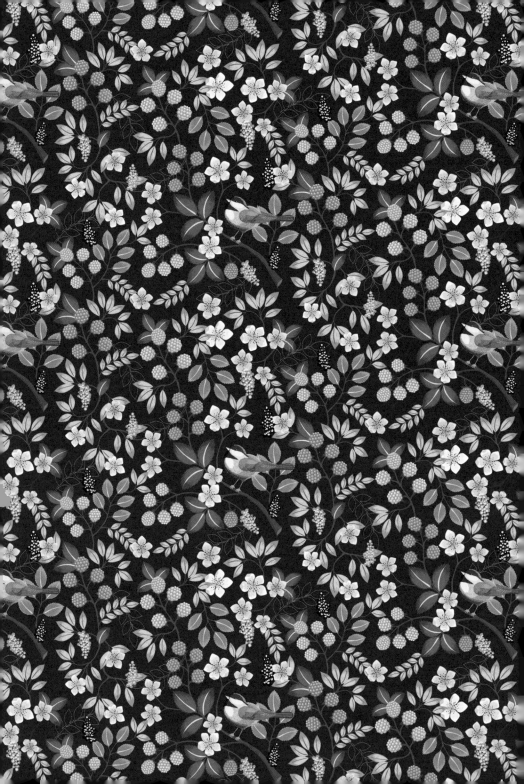

HERTHA'S HAUNT

1000AD

Our next journey is not as full of dread and danger as the last, in fact poetry will lead us to this place of peace – a sanctuary created for warriors fallen in battle. To lead us there I want to open with a verse from the *Poetic Edda*, a collection of Old Norse poems. A fitting charm to enable our journey as poetry was of utmost importance to the Norse figures we wish to chance upon. Odin himself is said to have brought the 'mead of poetry' to Asgard. But it is not Odin we hope to encounter...

Falcvanger's towers claim my song,

These to Freya's right belong;

Who chief presiding at each feast,

Appoints his place to ev'ry guest:

Half of the slain by her's possest,

But Odin daily claims the rest.

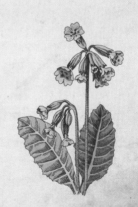

'The Song of Grimnir, XIV' from Icelandic Poetry

I want to wander back to the meadow we visited before, but this time to draw us back to a particular place, which I can connect us to with a plant. Let's seek out a cowslip (*Primula veris*), a plant once on the verge of extinction that now carries a more positive story – one of optimism and the potential for botanical life to return to places from which it had vanished. We will, however, seek it out in a garden, not in the wild. We do not wish to attract misfortune by harvesting this treasure in the meadow.

This bright, golden flower holds its magic within its old folk name 'key-plant.' In Scottish lore we trip over suggestions it may unlock the faerie queen's palace, and in more recent times it has been associated with St Peter and the gates to a Christian heaven.

But I reach for it now, knowing that this sleep-inducing, cough-relieving beauty, said to be able to soothe a temper and improve the mood, is also believed to be the key to Fólkvangr.

This may be the key we need to enter the next era which beckons us.

Fólkvangr is the field of the host, believed by some to be a palace within a meadow, hosted by the Norse goddess Freya and home to half of those slain in battle. She has the first pick of the warriors left on the field before Odin takes the rest to Valhalla. She rides on a chariot drawn by cats and uses the flower of the cowslip to open her gateway.

As we clench our floral cowslip key in our fist, we find ourselves sliding down the first root of Yggdrassil, the eternal Ash tree, which links the worlds. It is the tree of life and the gateway into Asgard. But it is not Freya we hope to encounter as our flower opens the doorway and we slide into another realm, it is her mother...

We are back in the meadow behind the castle where the two rivers meet. Strangely familiar, the meadow looks the same as last time, but the sounds and voices have altered. The season has not shifted since our last visit, it is still early July and the meadow is still humming with life. Peacock butterflies emerge from the nettles and carefully get a feel for their new wings. Swallows skim the air just above our heads, meadowsweet still softens the banks, and glittering red beetles adorn the cloud-like flowers of valerian (*Valeriana officianalis*), as a haze of hoverflies loiter above.

But more than that, the river's path has visibly shifted just a little. The pattern of houses on the opposite bank has changed. One tree has vanished and another oak sapling is now mature, its bark bulging with a weighty burr, the branches high above our heads. Beside it is a sturdy ash, one of its boughs keeping time, held within the flow of the rivers embrace.

The petrichor scented air vibrates warmly, humidity high, the grass still holds an essence of last night's thunderstorm. You run your fingers through the verdancy, and pink-tinged, white petals cover your hands as you brush the 'Cat's herb', valerian. The sleep-inducing dream-like scent said to be the secret lure that will in the future call the rats to follow the Pied

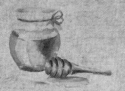

HERTHA'S LOVE PHILTRE: A MULLED HERBAL BEER

This herbal combination, whilst said to increase feelings of love, may also induce sleep... you have been warned!

Simmer a head of valerian flowers and three hop flowers in a cupful of good quality beer (a ginger beer made with natural ingredients is also ideal) for three minutes, then invite a lover to join you in sipping from the cup whilst warm.

If you wish to make an entirely non-alcoholic variant, then steep the herbs in a mugful of freshly boiled water for three minutes and then sweeten with honey.

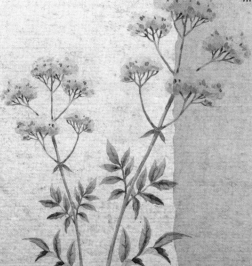

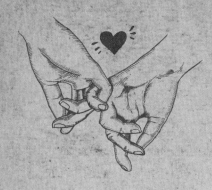

Piper away from Hamelin, drifts around you, lulling you into a languid torpor. Sure enough amongst the clouds of valerian are yellow cowslips, promising an opening through which to return, if we choose not to fully succumb to slumber.

As the wind clears the heady scent for a second, we realise we are not far enough into our time for this tale to have yet been told. We recognise a Nordic note to the voices hauling a small clinker-built rowing boat to shore and realise we are in the era when the seas were no boundary, but just a silver saline tidal road we shared with our Scandinavian neighbours.

HELD IN THE MOUTH, VALERIAN IS SAID TO CREATE TRUE LOVE FROM ONE KISS...

Or maybe just a sprig added to tea will do the trick, taking you back to Hertha's world where you can lie once again in a soft summer meadow with a lover and dream.

Valerian is said to bring peace and harmony if lovers argue, or maybe we'll dry the blooms to pop into a cloth bag to make a toy to lure cats we hope to convince to obey us, as Freya's do as they draw her chariot, in an unexpected act of obedience, long preceding that of the Pied Piper's Dance!

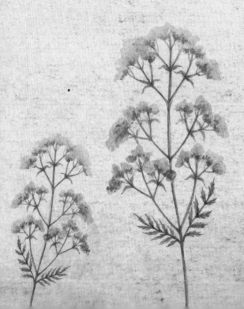

As you doze, you sense the soft tread of an animal approaching, hear a velvet muzzle crop the rich meadow nearby. You imagine words of ancient enchantment humming in the atmosphere and you lie half in a dream, half listening as you start to wonder what is happening to you.

Our meadow and valerian is holding you within its liminal world: part dream, part mythology.

Could that be the hand of Hertha – the Nordic goddess of nature whom we seek, mother to twins, Freya and Freyr, and said to have a special affinity with plants – gathering the fragrant stems as we rest on the earth? We try to avoid gazing at the figure, remembering the fate of those said to glimpse Hertha as she walks out of the waters of her home.

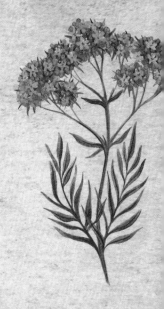

VALERIAN CAT TOY

Dried valerian has an aroma people either love or loathe. The scent of the flowers is more subtle than the ground root often used in herbal tea bags, but has a similar effect and is more sustainable to harvest. Gather a few stems in midsummer and hang them upside down to dry. Once dried they can be sewn into a fabric cat toy or tied into an old sock if you don't fancy sewing.

A valerian cat toy was once reputed to be an assured way of keeping a cat prone to wandering at home!

Although map archives suggest that the Pictish land of Fortiu may have covered land east from the Firth of Forth to Dalraida, and to Caithness in the north, the Danes are believed to have secured trade routes from York through the Firth of Forth to reach their other territories, the Western Isles and Dublin. As they traversed they took their familiar herbs and tested remedies, and they also took their ghosts and gods, their mythologies, legends, stories and beliefs. And they took Nerthus, the earth mother, and Njord – god of Vanir, protector of the sea, wind, fishing and wealth – her lover, divine partner or their other-self.

Nerthus was part of the soil, the land, the plants, the animals, holder of fertility and bringer of peace. Her name generously melds with the other 'terra mater' figures: the Germanic Ertha (or Hertha) and those haunting deities, who somehow seem familiar and have stories that blend with later Romantic fairy queens and classical huntress figures Diana and Artemis.

The image of Hertha with a crown of hops (*Humulus lupulus*), riding a stag and carrying the delicate valerian whip she uses to guide **the wild hunt,** connects her to the Pictish figure of Bride or Brigid. After all, these stories would have been woven together by storytellers at the time. There's a legend that tells of the **Cailleach** weaving her tapestry of the world, each charm being unravelled a little as she turns away, while Bride milked the fairy cattle of deer and made cheese, an apprentice in her cave, before eventually finding her own path after following a deer through the mist. I can easily imagine Hertha, or a similar missing mother figure of Scottish lore, wreathed in herbs, drawn by a hind, guiding Bride from the cave.

Maybe we have stumbled upon Hertha on our travels. Perhaps we have found her: casting dreams and drawing our thoughts to the earth as she leads the wild hunt.

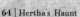

And now, the stag who brushes past us, with its bridle of hops leads us deeper into a world where sleep beckons. This could be the seductive world created by a love philtre of valerian and hops, the one Hertha is said to have used to entice her lovers, a love philtre that might lead even the most work-minded to contemplate idle afternoons spent lying in the arms of a lover in long meadow grass...

As the animal starts to move away, the spell breaks and you open your eyes, hoping to catch sight of a stag or maybe the figure of a woman with a certain timeless quality, but there is only the swaying of the cloud-like creamy plants of high summer to suggest anything has passed this way. Limbs still held in sleep, you gather a flower or two to carry with you as the spiral starts its work and once again we begin to slip forward in time.

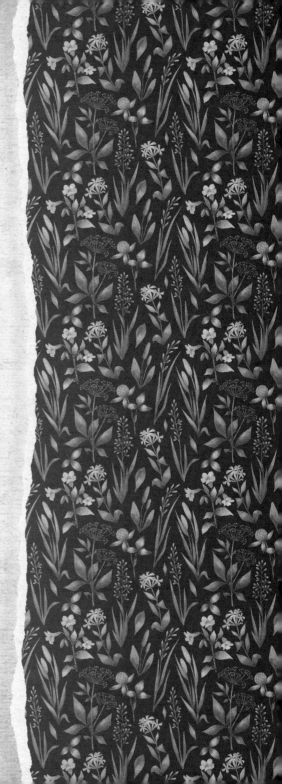

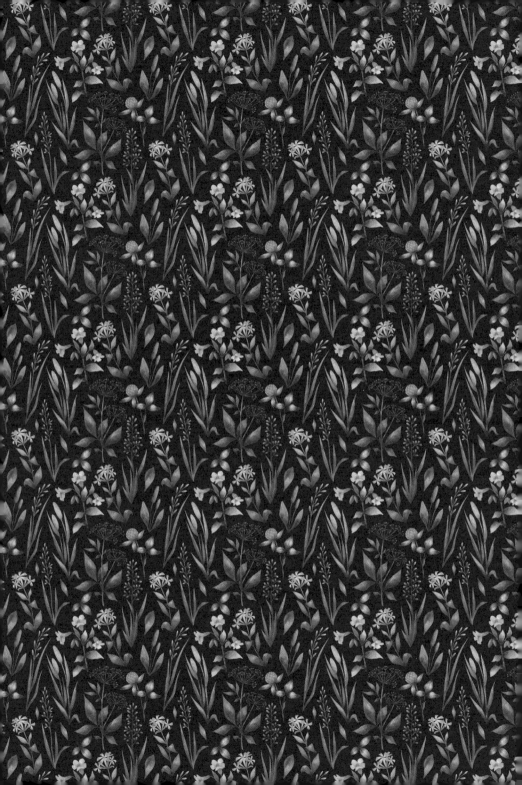

SPICES, FAIRYTALES AND PLAGUE

1367

With a jolt we find ourselves inside a large stone building, the walls hung with vivid, intricate tapestries. There are visitors arriving, voices talk of bringing spices and silks across land and sea, and stories have also travelled with these merchants. The seated spice traders are handed goblets of wine and plates of food by folk who must be the castle servants, who then encourage them to share tales of their journeys. These are people who have travelled far and seen many things. So as the sun sets, we find ourselves carried into a world shared from the Silk Road.

A French voice talks of a Syrian manuscript full of stories he has heard of in the *Bibliothèque Nationale de France*. Another man, opening a bundle of black peppercorns, says he has heard of these stories and laughs that the Lady of the castle could be the legendary slave girl of **Tawaddud**, outwitting every man with her knowledge of medicine, astrology and the practice of the healing arts. The room settles, sensing a traveller's story, one they have not heard before.

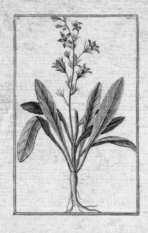

As the story begins there is a commotion as a young man enters the hall, breathless and frightened. He starts to tell the assembled group that his pregnant wife has been watching the garden of the old woman next door and now has a strong craving for parsley (*Petroselinum crispum*) and rapunzel roots (*Campanula rapunculus*). He is shaking because he has been to ask the old woman if he can have some of her plants for his wife, as she maybe needs the iron rich parsley or mineral rich parsnip flavoured rapunzel root. His wife is pale and tired and the baby is due soon. But the old woman has insisted the infant is given over into her charge in return for the herbs and vegetables the man has sought to borrow.

The assembled people start to whisper that the old woman, in her tower-like home, is not to be trusted. They say the loss of her own child has sent her mad and she is best avoided.

A woman looking over the spice-merchants' packages – redolent with the familiar aromas of cinnamon and ginger – departs and returns a few minutes later with a strikingly well-dressed woman. The richly attired noblewoman carries a baby in her arms and is calling out the names of the people she must remember to invite to her granddaughter's christening in the manner of someone who might at anytime become distracted by a more urgent task and forget to invite a vital guest. (If you listen carefully, you will hear the murmuring of hovering fairy godmothers...)

The people in the hall start to whisper, we gather that the lady is **Isobella McDuff**, Countess of Fife. She is the great grand-daughter of Edward the first of England and has succeeded to her father's lands. She has outlived three husbands, mothered three children, is courting husband number four, and currently refusing to hand over her lands to one of her brothers-in-law. She now looks after the lands and people, withstanding both plague and wars.

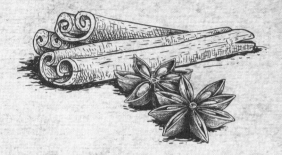

Her family line can be followed back to the legendary **Eleanor of Aquitaine** and, as is customary in her female line, she prides herself on her knowledge of healing plants and practices. She has read the works of **Trotula of Salerno** and **Hildegard of Bingen**, as her fore-mothers did, women who started hospitals and healing orders across Europe.

As the storyteller has paused, Isobella herself goes to the worried father-to-be and asks about his wife. She gives him a basket of **inulin**-rich, nourishing root vegetables, a bowl of dried nettle leaves, which she instructs him to add to soups with the vegetables to increase his wife's iron levels, and a handful of parsley, which she advises the woman should only take if she is certain the child is ready to arrive.

We sit and watch the room a little longer, following the lady as she goes to the kitchen with the woman who was buying the spices. Together they choose a pot containing peppercorns and cinnamon, raisins and green herbs in a good claret wine, and the pair decide this will help restore the new mother after the birth.

It would seem the old woman in the tower has a sad tale of her own, but she is best treated with caution as her own heartbreak has made her contrary. Maybe the storyteller will take her tale back on his travels and recount today's happenings, maybe they will find themselves in another story later on. But for now there is a baby to bring into the world and we begin to feel the patterns of time shift once more.

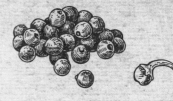

Vinegars

There will not be many of you, I suspect, who have not heard the legend from this period of the vinegar reputed to have been used by four thieves to help them avoid the plague and keep them healthy whilst they robbed the homes of the sick and dying. Legend has it that the original recipe was shared from a museum in Old Marseille, France, by Rene Maurice Gattefosse in his 1937 book, *Gattefossé's Aromatherapy*. It states:

Take three pints of strong white wine vinegar, add a handful of each of worm-wood, meadowsweet, wild marjoram and sage, fifty cloves, two ounces of cam-panula roots, two ounces of angelic, rosemary and horehound and three large measures of camphor. Place the mixture in a container for fifteen days, strain and express, then bottle. Use by rubbing it on the hands, ears and temples from time to time when approaching a plague victim.

Other versions of the story and variations of the recipe are widespread, but I'm not prepared to try them out to test their effectiveness! Nor quite honestly do I fancy daubing myself with the concoction and wandering around smelling of vinegar! So I've adapted the recipe to become one redolent with the valuable spices so prized in this era, a recipe that also owes thanks to herbalist **Rosemary Gladstar**'s tireless campaigning for the folk medicine 'fire cider', and not one to be branded and copyrighted.

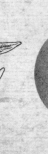

WARNING - some may find very hot spices and neat vinegar difficult. There are claims that some people on rare occasions have suffered oesophageal damage. So please use common sense and caution when taking this vinegar.

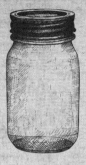
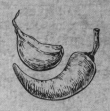

AROMATIC VINEGAR

This is a recipe that can be easily adapted to make the most of any surplus aromatic herbs, warming spices and antibiotic alliums, and is an easy and low-cost health supplement or a delicious additional ingredient to spice up a salad dressing.

In a glass or stoneware jar:

Add one finely chopped onion

Five cloves of crushed garlic (onions and garlic are common in cures and remedies from the Anglo-Saxon period onwards and are an effective remedy for several common diseases, in particular they are effective as an antibiotic against staphylococcal infections)

Twenty crushed black peppercorns

28g (1oz) chopped fresh herbs – the perfect blend combining immunity-enhancing effects and flavour are rosemary, thyme, sage and marjoram

Two finely chopped fresh chillies or a few dried (adjust to taste)

Cover in unpasteurised apple cider vinegar (labelled as 'with the mother', which indicates the live active agent that has beneficial properties), and firmly screw down

the lid. Leave to marinate for at least two weeks on a sunny windowsill. Shake daily and ensure the herbs and spices stay covered.

After straining, honey can be added to create what the ancient Greeks described as an 'oxymel'. This adds to its antimicrobial benefits and makes this type of vinegar a particularly delicious addition to salad dressings.

Apple cider vinegar enthusiasts recommend an egg-cupful in water before meals, but I like to take it if I feel run down or 'under the weather', or just add it to dressings and sauces.

WARNING: You could try washing in it like the four thieves did in the story, but I still feel that – while vinegar alone does have the ability to clean certain surfaces – one of *this* concoction's preventative effects was probably its power to repel people with its strong aroma!

Tonic Wine

A tonic wine is the perfect recipe to celebrate this era. The ascent of the barons had begun with William the Conqueror's arrival on British shores in 1066AD, after which they became more powerful than the English Saxon earls or Scottish thanes. Although wine had first been drunk in Britain during the Roman period, we know that the practice of viticulture was reduced with the arrival of the Vikings. It then increased again after King Alfred started to re-establish Christianity in England in around 878, coinciding with a beneficial warming in the climate, during which British vineyards flourished.

Whilst there were, we think, around 47 vineyards in England when the Normans invaded, and we can imagine a massive resurgence as the Norman aristocracy became the ruling demographic. This was not so much down to English wine growing but, for the first time ever, was due to trade. Henry II of England promoted trade routes between France and England, and the ruling barons from Anglo-French families (such as the family of Robert de Brus, later Robert the Bruce, King of Scotland) happily established the British taste for French wines.

We can also thank the Scottish kings for the spices that were so fashionable at the time – and a welcome addition to food and for health benefits. When the Scottish Royal Burghs were created they were granted a licence to trade spices, a lucrative business for seafaring families. The following recipe is a perfect nod to this moment in time.

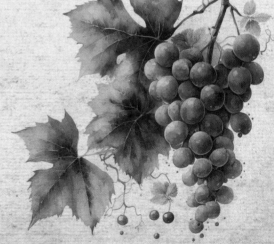

AN IRON TONIC

This tonic wine is based on a recipe told to me by one of my herbal teachers, the late Christopher Hedley. Rich in iron and other vitamins and minerals, it really is a homemade version of many of the liquid iron tonics on the market, designed to nourish and to be drunk daily in very small amounts (around 30ml/1fl oz).

Take a glass jar with a well-fitting lid. Add to the jar:

50g (1¾oz) sultanas

12 sulphur-free dried apricots, chopped

2 tbsp of dried nettle leaves. Only use the early top leaves of nettle. Pick and dry enough in the spring to last you throughout the year, as in late spring/early summer they develop **cystoliths** and can cause kidney problems. Later in the summer we can gather and use the seeds... but avoid the leaves!

Add a stick of cinnamon broken down in a pestle and mortar, a few corns of black pepper (worth more than its weight in gold in the 14th century), and a handful of rosehips (the vitamin C from the hips helps the body with the uptake of iron).

Top the jar up with good quality, preferably organic, red wine, making sure all the ingredients are well covered. Seal the jar and leave to infuse for two weeks, turning it twice daily.

Enjoy a small sherry-glassful every evening!

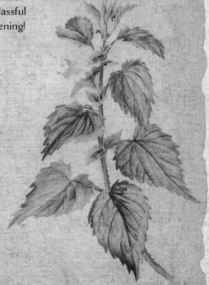

Note that the caffeine and tannin found in coffee and tea can reduce the body's ability to absorb iron, so should be avoided an hour before and after you take your tonic.

SPICES FOR WEALTH
AND HEALTH

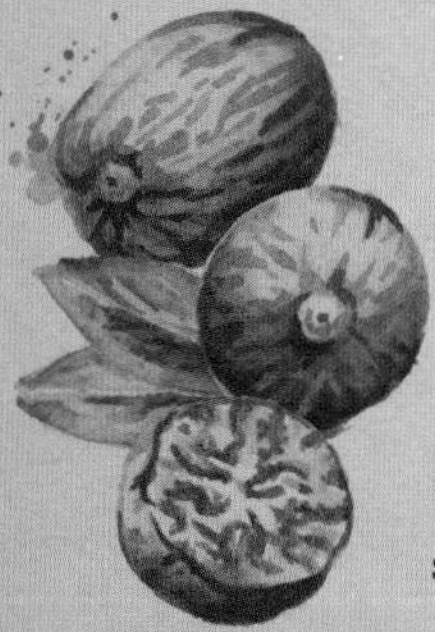

We are often told that various spices were once worth incredible sums. Pepper was worth over twice its weight in gold, with cloves, cinnamon and nutmeg achieving much higher prices. No doubt this influenced the use of certain spices in spells to attract wealth. Their strong aromatic scent also made them popular in plague deterrents.

In Chaucer's *Canterbury Tales* (1387–1400) the knight, Sir Thopas, who is in love with the Queen of Elfland, mentions nutmeg as an ingredient to add to ale or as an aromatic addition to a clothes coffer:

Ther spryngen herbes grete and smale,

The lycorys and the cetewale,

And many a clowe-gylofre

And notemuge to putte in ale,

Wheither it be moyste or stale,

Or for to leye in cofre.

We also know that the scent of nutmeg either as a 'fug' (burnt in a similar way to incense) or when worn as an amulet was, according to Chaucer's contemporaries, an accepted way to ward off plague. Priests often wore the spice in bags around their necks and one physician was said to pop a nutmeg in his mouth in the morning before treating patients in an attempt to avoid the pestilence.

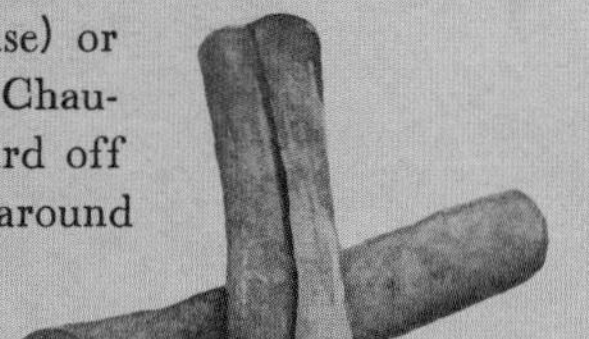

Spiced wine is being sipped, the air is becoming thick with something other than spices and incense. We are starting to twist back into the spiral, travelling forward into a world where we sense that tales of enchantment may soon be augmented with layers of fear. Things are about to become much darker.

Hold on to your protective charms, do not utter a word or pass judgement on things you see, because our time here is short and we cannot change the past. Keep your eyes down, remain unseen and do not challenge those who seek power, because the smoke no longer smells of cinnamon and nutmeg – the acrid smell of burning flesh lingers and there is a visceral sense of foreboding in the air.

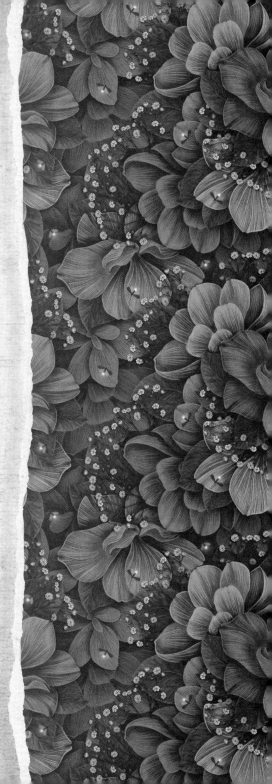

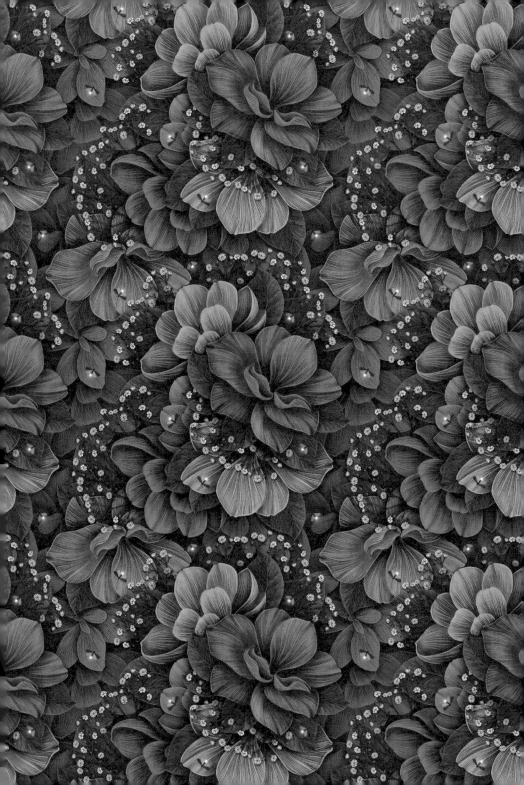

THE TRIALS

1597

As the time shifts pulse, we hear words again: prayer-like recitations, filled with palpable magic, words woven from the land, first in Gaelic then in translation. This is a yarrow charm, intoned as the plant is plucked in the hope to protect and strengthen the harvester. Again the words ground us and draw us to a place...

Buainidh mi an earr reidh,	I will pluck the yarrow fair,
Gum bu treuinide mo bhas,	That more brave shall be my hand,
Gum bu bhlathaide mo bheuil,	That more warm shall be my lips,
Gum bu ceumaide mo chas;	That more swift shall be my foot;
Gum bu h-eilean mi air muir,	May I an island be at sea,
Gum bu carraig mi air tir,	May I a rock be on land,
Leonar liom gach duine,	That I can afflict any man,
Cha leon duine mi.	No man can afflict me.

from Carmina Gadelica

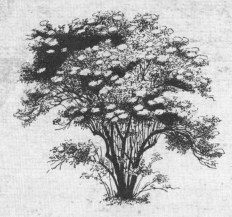

The meadow is familiar, but now the castle has grown, the village on the opposite bank has been replaced by a herd of cattle and a harbour now serves the castle.

A group of young women away from the crowds, are just within earshot, they whisper charms as they pick stalks of yarrow: guarding spells, woven around stalks kept for divining, the flowers strewn in baskets to make remedies for colds and wound-healing balms.

The ominous figure of a man of religion appears and the girls' whispering turns to pious talk and deferential words, the stalks clasped into skirt folds, innocent flower-heads piled into baskets.

A now familiar murmuring comes, seemingly from within the shivering branches of an elder tree (*Sambucus nigra*), planted, protectively, outside a stone dairy building – maybe the aroma from the leaves is deterring flies – its branches laden with berries and drying cheesecloths. It seems to whisper of daemons and familiars...

There seems to be the suggestion of a figure in the trunk of the tree – the Elder Mother is near. Because elder is home to a witch, she may protect you, as she does the back door of this stone building. The front door is being protected by the red berried rowan (*Sorbus aucuparia*).

A woodsman approaches, a youth tags along carrying a bow saw. We watch, resting a few feet away, by a stand of purple flowering mint

(*Mentha spp.*) and listen as the master tells his apprentice to recite before cutting, the words of a traditional charm to humour the spirit of the elder:

'Old friend, dear wife, give me some of thy wood and I will give thee some of mine when I grow into a tree'

...explaining that to break or cut a branch from the elder will upset the witch, the creature, the mother, to whom the tree is home.

He explains how the soft pith will come out easily from the branch to fashion a chanter, a pipe to practice a dancing air upon. A pipe gifted from a witch, he laughs, adding that it will protect from one more malevolent, as long as it isn't played on All Hallow's Eve. The master tries scaring his apprentice, with a glint in his eye, explaining it may summon **The Wild Hunt** and he will get stolen away if he doesn't heed this advice.

As they leave the girls walk forward, in turn asking permission and thanking the tree, as they gather the ripening berries and add them to their baskets. They talk of the recent visit from the king and of the resulting obsessions from the church, now intent on routing out witches.

Care must be taken. The dairy, they gossip, has reduced its use of lady's bedstraw (*Galium verum*) as the colour-enhancing, curdling agent to make cheese. The dairymaids are afraid of being accused of stealing the cream from a neighbour's cattle if the golden flowers produce too rich a colour.

The midwife is taking every precaution, working long hours and gathering all possible herbal remedies in preparation for the cold dark hours of winter. She is wary of losing a mother or child and being accused of taking the devil's pay.

They still divine with the stalks of yarrow (*Achillea millefolium*) – the chance of foreseeing a marriage or charming a future too beguiling to miss – but now they must be cautious. They make fever and flu relieving elixirs to distract from the games that accompany their cooking, because these are the days of daemonolgy. The king has written of the women who conjure storms, who court familiars, of succubi and lycanthropes. These are dangerous days and there are fires to come...

To Fight the Flames of Fevers and Flu

The girls we have met on our journey are gathering yarrow, elder and mint. Earlier in the year when the elder is in flower, the blossom along with flowering tops of yarrow and mint leaves, would be dried (or used fresh), as a diaphoretic, fever relieving tea (known commonly as YEP or EPY tea, or occasionally 'gypsy tea').

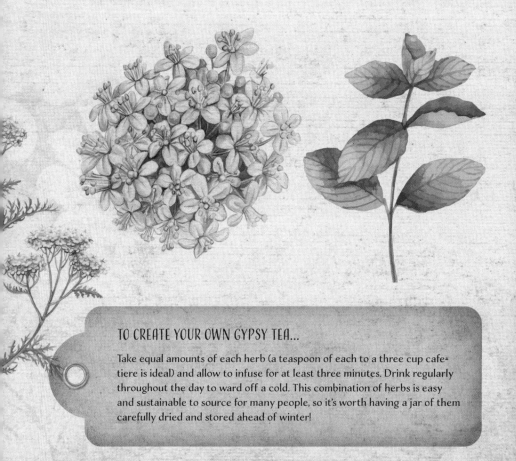

TO CREATE YOUR OWN GYPSY TEA...

Take equal amounts of each herb (a teaspoon of each to a three cup cafetiere is ideal) and allow to infuse for at least three minutes. Drink regularly throughout the day to ward off a cold. This combination of herbs is easy and sustainable to source for many people, so it's worth having a jar of them carefully dried and stored ahead of winter!

Yarrow flowers late enough to gather with elderberries at the summer's end, and mint is one of the most prolific soft herbs in the garden, easily found in the wild until the first frosts, so I also like to create a yarrow and mint infused elderberry elixir. It can be used to ward off end-of-year colds and flu. But beware because just a few years from now, collecting yarrow will become one of the recognised signs of practicing witchcraft. In the 1590s the whispers are already getting louder. Collecting yarrow in a ritualised manner is to be one of the accusations made of Elspeth Roach, who will be convicted of witchcraft on Orkney in 1616. So as you gather the plants to prepare your elixir, be mindful of the freedom now afforded to you and spare a thought for those who have not been able to cure their own ailments in times past for fear of persecution.

The word 'elixir', which really resonates with winter days when magical things seem so close, owes its origins to the years predating the late sixteenth century. It is associated with the **philosopher's stone** of alchemists, promising a cure from disease and prolonging life. In the 1590s it was the term used for a strong tonic or alcohol-based remedy. A blend of honey and alcohol is particularly effective at drawing the active constituents out of plants. If you wish to avoid alcohol, then vinegar will act as a reasonable alternative.

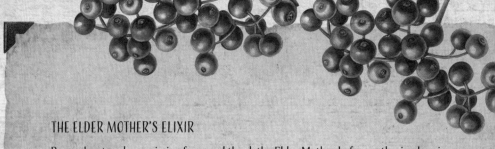

THE ELDER MOTHER'S ELIXIR

Remember to ask permission from and thank the Elder Mother before gathering berries.

Take a handful of washed and gently dried, fresh yarrow flowers and a few leaves.

Add a handful of fresh mint. Including a few flowers in with the leaves is good.

Chop both together finely.

Pour into a sterilised glass jar with a screw-top lid, and add the fruit from ten heads of ripe elderberries (be careful to remove all stalks as these can cause an upset stomach).

Spoon in four tablespoons of local honey and cover with whisky.

Shake well, then place on a sunlit window ledge. Allow the elixir to infuse for two or three weeks, shaking the jar regularly to keep the ingredients covered and blending.

Take a teaspoon up to three times a day at the first sign of a cold or flu.

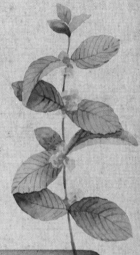

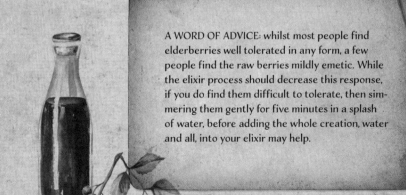

A WORD OF ADVICE: whilst most people find elderberries well tolerated in any form, a few people find the raw berries mildly emetic. While the elixir process should decrease this response, if you do find them difficult to tolerate, then simmering them gently for five minutes in a splash of water, before adding the whole creation, water and all, into your elixir may help.

There's an traditional Irish saying that goes, 'anyone can lose their hat to a fairy wind', and a fairy wind this must be, for there is something elemental about the gusts.

I think it's time to add another protective charm, another amulet to our collection. Before we are whisked further forward in time, I suggest you find a piece of iron – something simple, lost or discarded, like a time worn nail, an antique key, or maybe a horseshoe. Then pour a dish of cream or cut a piece of cake and bring that too, because gifts are well regarded where we are about to go.

The burning days have not yet ended, but now there is something else we may need protection from: something that is hidden, repelled by iron, but desirous of cake! Something we may need to respect and stay on our guard around, especially if we wish to return to our own time...

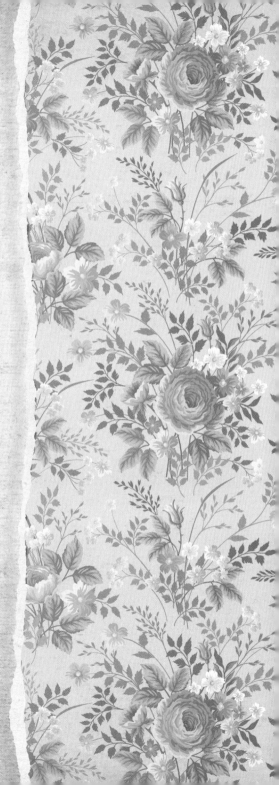

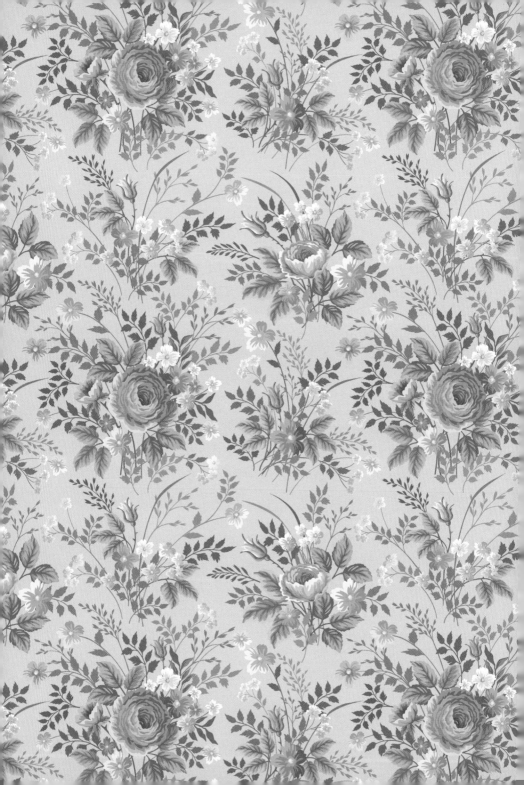

HUSH, YOU MAY KNOW TOO MUCH...

1692

If you feel you may be seeing people not-quite-there, an ethereal presence shifting in and out of your peripheral vision, you are not alone...

For we may have slipped through time again into the company of the first person to translate the bible into Gaelic. A minister who believed in many things beyond the boundaries of his **kirk**. A man who was intent on proving and then exploring the world of the sidh or fae, the good folk, in part due to his studies as a folklorist, in part to prove to the atheists of the time – intent on discrediting the church – that if the faerie folk existed, then so must angels and devils. His aim: to unveil a cohort of sentient life-forms, parallel to humanity, but each realm of beings subtly different in make-up.

In time, we will become acquainted with The Reverend Robert Kirk of Aberfoyle – a man who famously appeared one last time as an apparition. He will whisper his story to us soon, but first we need to take stock of our surroundings.

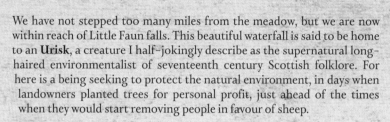

We have not stepped too many miles from the meadow, but we are now within reach of Little Faun falls. This beautiful waterfall is said to be home to an **Urisk**, a creature I half-jokingly describe as the supernatural long-haired environmentalist of seventeenth century Scottish folklore. For here is a being seeking to protect the natural environment, in days when landowners planted trees for personal profit, just ahead of the times when they would start removing people in favour of sheep.

The waterfall descends from a hill, surrounded by hills. Hills clad in protective rowan, cleansing birch, Douglas fir and Scots pine, their evergreen needles symbolising longevity and immortality. The boulders along the path of the stream are covered in soft emerald swathes of moss. We can see a village and a modest church at the foot of the hill, and across from the village, just beyond the church, sits a small regular dome shaped hill, its shape incongruous alongside the more rugged ice-age formed landscape.

Back in our own time, we will have heard the voices of the evidence-driven experts say that these even, somewhat symmetrical, hills are often the sites of iron age hill forts, or sometimes **Pictish** earth works. They might be village sites, but sometimes there are no other clues, just a strange semi-sphere, rising from a field. If it's topped by an oak, an ash and a thorn... well then, it's fair to ponder that it might indeed be a fairy hill.

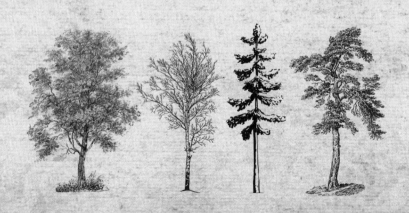

This one at the edge of Robert Kirk's parish is Doon hill, and as we follow the learned man past the village and the **kirk** towards it, we realise he is taking copious notes, observing his surroundings. It is twilight, and he is remarking to himself as he writes that this is the best time of the day to see them. That they are astral, changeable beings and of a nature a little like condensed clouds. He stops and looks to a field of oats, muttering that they steal the corn like the crows and mice. But he also concedes that some of their ilk, the brownies, help around the house, undertaking domestic duties, and that while they may steal the corn when doing so, they may also leave the ricks more copious than they were before.

He writes that the **fairy howe** by his church is believed by the superstitious of his parish to be where the souls of their predecessors dwell. It's a spot dedicated by the church and its graveyard to receive the departed, thus becoming a fairy hill. For at this time the Reverend Robert Kirk is writing, not a bible on this occasion, but a treatise on the 'Secret Commonwealth', the world of elves, fauns and fairies.

He must be near the end of his work as he leaves a full notebook, stuffed with extra pieces of paper, on the table of the manse house by the church, and starts to walk towards the domed hill. As we also begin to ascend, we notice hazelnuts ripening on the boughs of small trees and note the scent of wild thyme as our legs brush through the undergrowth. Something compels us to gather a few stems, a nut or two as we go... and we lose sight of the minister as he continues upwards along a twisting path.

There is something enchanted about this place, so we stop to share stories of folk who have encountered the fae, such as Thomas A' Rhymer, of Ercildoune in the Borders, who shared a beautiful sonnet with the fairy queen and was rewarded with an apple containing the gift of prophecy. Although, for his trouble, he lost seven years in the mortal world. Or the farmhand from the village of Killin in the Perthshire highlands, who fell asleep on a fairy knowe and when he awoke at sunset saw a couple cooking, though they didn't see him. He accidentally got a speck of hot porridge from their pot in his eye and could see the fairies from then on... until he saw **The Wild Hunt** pass through the town and the ethereal beings realised they were visible to him and put out his eye. Or the lady who conjured an enchanted dress of fairy green so as to capture the heart of a lover and who fell at her wedding never to return, her grave now marked by a stone that **birls** at midnight on hallowe'en. A shiver goes through our group. The moon has risen, darkness envelops the land and we are talking too much of the good folk... maybe we should hush.

As morning arrives, we are awoken by a clamour. The minister has been discovered inert on the hilltop. Whispers go round that he knew too much, he has been stolen away by the fae.

As the weeks pass the minister is buried, a stone marking his grave, but then he appears as the banns are read for his cousin's wedding. He moves away from any embrace and tells his relative that he has been taken away by the good folk, but there is one chance to restore him. He will appear at the wedding and the cousin must throw his dirk, a ceremonial knife, at his form. Freeing him from the spell.

Sure enough a few weeks later, the minister appears again, but the cousin cannot throw a knife at the man he values as a friend and Robert Kirk is never seen again. His body so the story goes is not within his grave. Instead the coffin is said to be filled only with stones...

The Reverend's work is gathered up and locked in a wooden box... we know the family passes it on, through the generations, until one day, it will be published – the work of a man who knew too much and was stolen away by the fae.

There is something I need to tell you, something that happened back in our own time, or at least not so very long ago. I was gathering tales and memories of plant lore from older folk in rural Stirlingshire, not far from this village of Aberfoyle, when an old lady – she was 94 at the time – told me that she had heard from her grandmother of an ointment that would enable you to see into the magical world of the sidh.

She remembered some of the ingredients, but not all of them. The full list had been written down and passed on through generations until a learned man had bought it from a relative and taken it away to his museum in England. I started to look for this mysterious recipe, and eventually found reference to it being in the archive of the Ashmolean Museum in Oxford. Serendipitously, I was then invited to Oxford, to the Ashmolean itself, to share a herbal storytelling workshop as part of a new exhibition. The opportunity to see the infamous recipe first hand had presented itself!

Oxford was beautiful, the museum incredible, the exhibition breathtaking – a fascinating blend of art and history. It all felt rather magical, but although I mentioned the recipe to many people who worked in the museum, no one had heard of it and we couldn't find where it might be kept.

As I went to leave at the end of the day, I was tapped on the shoulder by an elderly gentleman. His face was rendered bark-like, lined like an oak, by the twisting of time. He was dressed in a uniform that seemed to be from another era. He explained he might know where the recipe was and led me to a lift, pressing a combination of buttons, exiting into an underground cellar, with a high arched ceiling, festooned with cobwebs. At the end of the cellar was a room, and in the room was a cast-iron box, which the man unlocked.

There was just one piece of paper inside.

Smiling the man unrolled it – it was written in the handwriting of another time and dated 1600. An ointment to see the fae.

I had a notebook and he nodded his assent, permission to write it down.

When we got back to the back door of the museum, and as I went to gather up my bag, he must have turned and gone back inside, as he seemed to have melted away.

I went in to thank Dr Sarah, who had invited me along to the work-shop, and I asked about the man and the cellar. She just looked at me oddly and said she didn't know who he was, and that she had looked again but still didn't know about the recipe, or where it might be. However, if I thought I now had it, then she was sure I could share it.

So I share it with you, I trust if you've read this far, then you will know how to use it carefully!

Do not expect a counter-bought modern ointment – this is more of an emulsion. If you grind the ingredients down they will help to blend the oil and water. I will not translate it, but share it with you as I wrote it down...

A LOTION TO ENABLE ONE TO SEE THE FAIRIES

Take a pint of sallet oyle and put it into a vial glasse;

and first wash it with rose-water and marygolde water.

The flowers to be gathered towards the east.

Wash it till the oyle becomes white, then put it into the glasse,

and then put thereto the budds of hollyhock,

the flowers of marygolde,

the flowers or toppes of wild thyme the budds of young hazle, and the thyme must be gathered near the side of a hill where fairies use to be;

and take the grasse of a fairy throne; then all these put into the oyle in the glasse and sette it to dissolve three dayes in the sunne and then keep it for thy use.

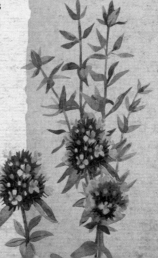

It does make a lovely lotion. I have myself used the sun infusing method for the following flowers: hollyhocks (*Alcea sp.*), which in the Victorian language of flowers were associated with fecundity and ambitions obtained; pot marigolds (*Calendula officinalis*), which have antifungal properties; wild thyme (*Thymus polytrichus*), which is antibacterial; roses (*Rosa sp.*), which smell sweet and tone the skin; buds of hazelnut (*Corylus avallana*), which are nourishing. I then strained the emulsion and used a little between the brows in the third eye area and the rest as a lovely hand lotion. I have also tried grinding the botanicals up in a pestle and mortar first, then leaving them in the ointment as the original recipe is not clear whether they should be removed or not.

Finding the ingredients of course may take time, research will need to be done. I have a few words of advice: to find a fairy knowe, listen to the stories of your area, where there is a hill there will be a local story. Many guides say that fairy knolls are topped by an oak, an ash and a thorn, so maybe that will give you a clue as to where to start.

Remember that for the 'grasse from a fairy throne' you may well need to do some guess-work!

I found the tell-tale shape of a seat on the top of a certain legendary hill, encased within a ring of mushrooms. Could this have been a fairy throne? I was mindful of the old advice about collecting and gathering all plants: 'don't take too much and leave a thank you'. Traditionally fairies like a glass of milk and a piece of cake... but that's another story!

I will not reveal whether or not I have seen the fae as that would seem unwise. But if you see them, remember the rules:

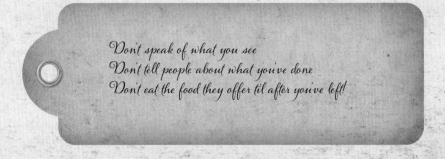

Don't speak of what you see
Don't tell people about what you've done
Don't eat the food they offer til after you've left!

Maybe it's safe to take your own notes and hold the story close. Write it on nettle paper, fold it in a piece of silk and lock it in an iron box. Save your tale of the fae to hand on to one of your family, your own family fairy story to treasure.

TO INFUSE AN OIL WITH POT MARIGOLD

If you do decide to make the mixture to help you see the fae, then you may need to know how to cold-infuse an oil with pot marigold (*Calendula officinalis*, the 'marygolde' in the original recipe). For the 'salate oyl' mentioned I would use a locally sourced cold-pressed oil. In Scotland for example, rapeseed oil is easily found and is a beautiful golden yellow. Almond or sunflower oil are also ideal options.

Take the clean, fresh (or dried) flowers of pot marigold and fill a jar completely.

Cover with the oil, making sure all the flowers are submerged.

Tightly fasten the lid and place on a sunny windowsill for 2-3 weeks.

Strain the mixture through a muslin or jelly bag, making sure you squeeze the last potent drops of oil out of the plant matter.

Repeat with new flowers and the original infused oil.

This infusion also makes a wonderful massage oil for dry skin and mild dry eczema. It has anti-fungal benefits, making it effective for some fungal conditions.

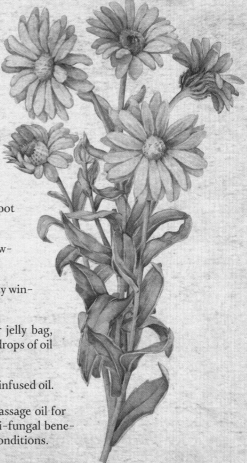

TO MAKE ROSEWATER

One of the best-known home remedies – even if you don't realise you almost certainly know it already! You probably made flower water as a child...

Do you remember picking petals and leaving them in water to make 'perfume'? Well, that is a basic rosewater.

Fill a jar with petals of a scented rose, any species (wild or cultivated) will do as long as it is unsprayed.

Cover with filtered water, shake well and leave overnight.

Strain and use.

Will keep for a couple of days in the fridge.

Rosewater also makes an effective skin toner, having rejuvenating and toning effects.

As a final warning, remember the tale of the midwife, who is asked by a stranger to help his wife who is in labour. He takes her to a cottage she has never seen before. She assists a woman birthing, but when the child is born the couple say they must leave, and they ask her to care for the child. The midwife feels she has no choice as they must leave quickly. All she is left with is a carved wooden cradle, a blanket, food and a sweet-scented green liquid, which she is told to apply daily to the baby's face. The couple impress upon her that she is never to use it on herself.

The weeks go past and the mid-wife does as she's been asked. Food is always provided – by whom she does not know – so she stays and happily cares for the child. Until one day a bee disturbs her as she's applying the green lotion to the baby, the heady pollen makes her sneeze and she accidentally gets oint-ment on her face. Suddenly she sees that the room is just a cave and the child is no earthly baby but a strange creature, laughing at magical ethereal beings that lurk in the corners of the cave.

The midwife leaps up realising how long she's been there, and goes to leave. But she is trapped in a subterranean world, and there is no way out.

There she spends the rest of time, happy and well cared for, but never able to return to the land of mortals.

So use the lotion carefully...

SIMPLE THYME TEA

Thyme tea has been used to ward off respiratory in-fections, coughs and colds for centuries.

Take three sprigs of fresh thyme flowers and leaves (or a teaspoon of dried thyme – the shop bought stuff is fine if that's what you have to hand), and place in a mug, Pour over freshly boiled water.

Allow to steep for three to five min-utes, then strain.

Add a teaspoon of honey and the juice of half a lemon.

Take at the first suggestion of a cold, until it goes away.

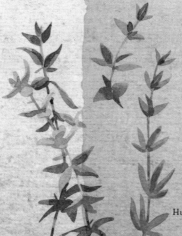

A GLIMPSE OF A ROSY FUTURE?

'O My Luve is like a red, red rose that's newly sprung in June...' wrote Rabbie Burns in 1794, though his song was based on a much earlier traditional piece. But beyond its familier link with romance, the rose also has been associated with seeing other beings as well as fairies...

Local variants of this charm occur across the British Isles, but the version I was taught by an old lady in rural Perthshire (back in my late teens) works like this:

Pluck a red rose (newly sprung in June) at midnight on the nearest full moon to Midsummer.

Wrap it in a piece of clean white cloth, which must belong to you.

Put it somewhere safe until **Hogmanay**.

When the bells announcing the new year ring, unwrap the rose...

...and an apparition of your future spouse will appear and snatch the rose away!

We, however, can leave it would seem as my stories are now done. We realise the world has begun to shift once more and we are travelling on through time. A new era beckons. But maybe we'll take a thyme tea with us, just in case anyone coughs or sneezes and accidentally rubs a little fairy lotion in their eyes!

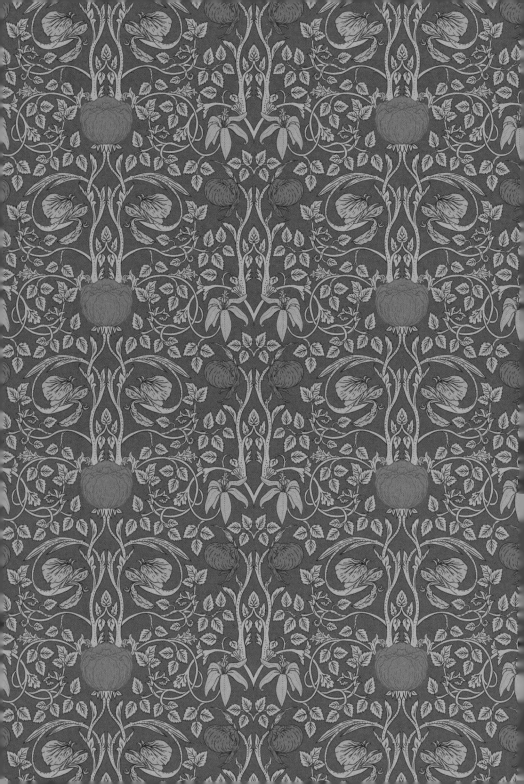

THE VERY CURIOUS HERBAL

1730

We are nearing the final flourish of our spiral back through time, but before I allow you to access the words that will send you back to where you began, I want to take you on a journey to the place I was born. Aberdeen is a city that's always had an air of rebelliousness, a history of innovation and of standing up for what it believes in, determined to change things for the better.

This is a granite-graced, silver city with a reputation for its ability to endure; a place that takes intuitive, inspired steps to explore, making the most of the twists and turns life offers it.

At the beginning of the eighteenth century (some 270 years before my arrival), in the Aberdeen that Elizabeth Blachrie – the woman to whom I'm about to introduce you– was born, rum had recently become available. It was introduced by sailors familiar with the North Sea, which borders the city, who would have constantly brought in new tastes and new ideas. However, the real innovations in the city run to the more prosaic but no less vital street lighting, road sweeping, and also the letting up somewhat on the previous century and half of witch burning for a wee bit... possibly to give itself a rest for just long enough to become the heartland of the Jacobite rebellion.

But more about that will reveal itself shortly...

I first met Elizabeth in the pages of a book held in the hauntingly beautiful environs of the Royal College of Physicians and Surgeons in Glasgow. Whilst the library does contain the copy of Mrs Blackwell's (as she is to become) *A Curious Herbal: 500 cuts of the most useful plants, which were at the time used in the practice of physick,* it does not contain on any rote or list, honorary or otherwise that I know of, the name of Alexander Blackwell, with whom Elizabeth Blachrie eloped shortly before his medical credentials were questioned.

This book, *A Curious Herbal,* has fallen open on a careful study of larch (*Larix decidua*), a plant I immediately reach for as a Bach flower remedy, an essence I use to promote confidence in one's creative abilities. The picture draws us into this book, offering us the chance to meet Elizabeth in her extraordinary time.

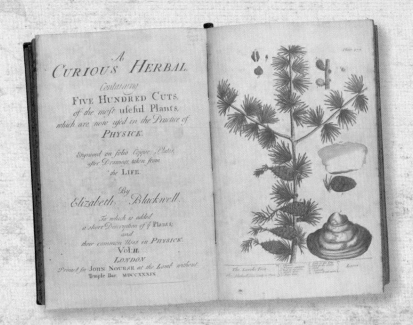

She is married to Alexander, who is by all accounts a good student, excelling at languages, but prone to being – how shall I put this? – a bit of a blagger. Maybe that's part of the draw for Elizabeth, as it's clear that they are both charismatic, intelligent and ambitious people, who know their own minds. Although, while good decision making is not Alexander's forte, Elizabeth is clearly made of a different mettle.

I suspect a little passion is also at play because passion, perseverance and a deep love of plants are clearly hard-wired into Elizabeth's nature.

Having escaped from the fallout of Alexander's exploits back in Aberdeen, the couple have made their way to London and have used her funds to set Alexander up in a printing business (I suspect the English law of coverture, which did not bind couples in Scotland, has been steadfastly ignored by the forward-thinking Blackwells!). Now Elizabeth has quite suddenly found herself alone in London with a young son, her husband incarcerated in a debtor's jail, his reputation once again in question.

She might be forgiven for upping and heading home to her parents, living as she does in a time when middle-class women do not go out and work, but instead she has taken to studying the plants and learning from the collectors and gardeners at Chelsea Physic Garden.

Elizabeth has had her first taste of a fresh orange within the walls of this garden, its sharp sweet acidity bringing refreshed positivity and new ideas to her mind. She is highly regarded by Sir Hans Sloane, the director Isaac Rand, and head gardener Phillip Miller, who are duly impressed at her suggestion that a comprehensive new herbal is needed, with accurate representations of the plants that they revere.

She has proposed a feat which many folk assure us, had never before been undertaken by a woman. To create and publish a complete herbal featuring life-like illustrations of the plants in use by apothecaries of the time.

As I muse over her work, each plant immediately identifiable, many rarely seen in the British Isles by anyone other than the elite travellers and the wealthier apothecaries, it strikes me that there were very few herbals created before this by anyone – man or woman – of this magnitude. Books that offered identifiable pictures and concise, accessible notes on plants sourced from around the world were scarce, and this was made at a pivotal point in history, when such a herbal had vast implications. Here are cacao, coffee, tamarind, turmeric, tomatoes and cucumbers, plants rarely seen – new exotics in this time of enlightenment – alongside the familiar hedgerow plants sought by the skeely-wife, the cunning folk, and the everyday people turning to hedgerows for remedies, plants such as dandelion, thistles, sloes and hawthorn.

The tastes of Africa, the Americas and India are only just being discovered at this point in history. This is no small work, unique not only because its illustrator was a woman, but a significant piece, that we should view in the context of the incredible, often difficult time in which Elizabeth lives.

I search further, baffled as I challenge what I'd been told back in our time, that the words of the herbal were written by her husband from his cell at Highgate. I see Elizabeth spending so much time at this leading physic garden, home to the Worshipful Society of Apothecaries, a place where she has friends and has learnt from doctors, gardeners and plant collectors, a place with a library of herbals. I come to realise that the claims that Alexander wrote this book have no substance and show little consideration of the circumstances or aptitudes of either of the Blackwells!

Elizabeth shares insights into the potential for the then exotic tomato, its Latin name *Lycopodium persica* is literally translated as 'the wolf peach'. But it is not yet fixed as Linnaus is still to create his categorisations, and Elizabeth calls it 'the love apple'. She suggests it is eaten as a salad ingredient, something we know her friends the Sloanes had learnt from Spanish migrants in the Americas. She informs her readers of this, in a time when many people in Britain still studiously avoid the acidic red fruit, terrified by the northern European story that it is used by witches to turn their enemies into werewolves. They firmly believe it is safest kept as a decorative plant, placing it on mantelpieces, where they think it helps attract wealth to the home.

Elizabeth shares instructions that coffee, a fashionable drink at this time, being shared by the era's most forward of thinkers in the new and aspirational coffee shops, can be used 'to relieve a phlegmatic disposition', energising she declares, as the caffeine blocks the adenosine receptors.

Her innovative work is reaching a wide audience, sharing knowledge at an affordable rate, published episodically in pamphlet form, in a time when healing practices are becoming more and more regulated; just after the last of those accused of witchcraft have been burnt.

We spot that fairy stories are no longer the valued learning resource they once were, no longer a vital way of discovering the healing arts. We stop mutely and listen as we hear one last story begin, it is being shared by an old storyteller, a woman with long, thick hair, greying at the temples but not truly indicating her years. She bids us to be careful not to brush past the Noedl, Naughty Man's Plaything, Scaddie, Hoky-poky, Devil's Leaf, Heg-beg, Stingers... Nettles and adds if they do skim our ankles just remember:

Nettle in, Dock out, Dock rubs Nettle out.

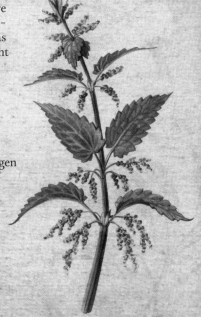

Nettle (*Urtica dioica*) is so full of seeds as late summer arrives. I harvested jars full last year, before we embarked on our journey, and remember encountering them in the back of the cupboard as spring was just emerging – the air still smelling of snow, sunlight just beginning to lick the earth, bringing with it the fresh taste of new nettle growth.

I remember walking along the water's edge today, past the **kirk** along meadowsweet-lined paths, gathering nettle seeds as swans flew overhead.

Nettle seeds are so energising, a natural adaptogen they've helped me through the moves and shifts of the last year and I confess I feel a kindred soul in this plant, one that I'm sure Elizabeth Blackwell would have loved too: bolshy, bossy but benevolent plant of Aries that it is.

The COMPLEAT

HOUSEWIFE:
OR,
Accomplish'd Gentlewoman's
COMPANION:
Being a COLLECTION of upwards of Six
Hundred of the moſt approved RECEIPTS in

COOKERY,	CAKES,
PASTRY,	CREAMS,
CONFECTIONARY,	JELLIES,
PRESERVING,	MADE WINES,
	CORDIALS.

them with your fingers before they are bak'd ; let
the oven be ready for them against they are done ;
be careful the oven does not colour them.

To make the thin Dutch Bisket.

TAKE five pounds of flour, and two ounces of
çarraway-seeds, half a pound of sugar, and
something more than a pint of milk ; warm the
milk, and put into it three quarters of a pound of
butter ; then make a hole in the middle of your
flour, and put in a full pint of good ale-yeast ;
then pour in the butter and milk, and make these
into a paste, and let it stand a quarter of an hour
by the fire to rise ; then mould it, and roll it into
cakes pretty thin ; prick them all over pretty
much, or they will blister ; so bake them a quarter
of an hour.

To make an ordinary Seed Cake.

TAKE six pounds of fine flour, rub into it : a
thimble-full of caraway feeds finely beaten,
and two nutmegs grated, and mace beaten ; then
beat a quart of cream hot enough to melt a pound
of butter in it, and when it is no more than blood-
warm, mix your cream and butter with a pint of

... for
... ous

... e Year.

... ily RECEIPTS
... Ointments, and
... roved Efficacy
... is, Sores &c.
... ate Families, or
... neficient to their

... s ; not in any

... Golden Buck,
... treet. 1739.

Seek out nettles, gather their seeds, or find a handful of new leaves and add them to a potage. Watch how they reclaim neglected sites, healing our waste, turning middens into minerals. Note how they offer relief from allergies to pollen or maybe to feathers...

The soft ripe seeds are full of strength, gifting fortitude when needed to complete a task. Elizabeth Blackwell noted nettle seeds' value for shortness of breath, a testimony to its rejuvenating nature.

Having gathered a handful of nettle seeds, quietly thinking by the River Tweed years ago, I had laid them out to dry on a cloth made of silken soft, knitted nettle fibres. I then cast the seeds into a biscuit inspired by a recipe found in Eliza's Smith's *The Compleat Housewife* of 1736 – tying in a gift of spelt for the Roman goddess of agriculture, Ceres. Now I invite you to eat one and cast your mind back to your own childhood. Maybe you remember the story of the girl who weaves nettle shirts for her brothers to save them from being swans, trapped within an enchantment. It's a story that seems to be riven into the DNA of many folks fascinated by plants... but one that if you don't know it, I will tell you if you find a way to listen, a story whispered across the spirals of time.

Nettles are just one example of the way in which our attitude to plants changes over time. In Elizabeth's day fabric is often made from nettles, retted down, becoming soft and linen-like in texture. Paper for important documents is made from nettle fibre, and it is rightly considered a vital nutritionally rich ingredient in the early days of Spring when our bodies crave fresh green iron-rich food after the strength-sapping cold of winter.

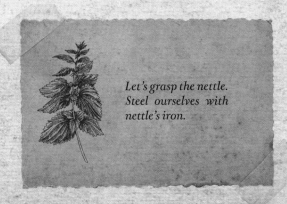

Let's grasp the nettle.
Steel ourselves with
nettle's iron.

NETTLE HAIR TONIC

Take five tablespoons of dried nettles. Collect plenty and dry in the
oven overnight after you've cooked,
spreading them out on a tray to
allow air to circulate. Turn them
and let them dry slowly to protect
the constituents. Or leave for a few
days in a warm, dry place, checking
and turning them to prevent mould.
Alternatively use a handful of fresh
nettle leaves.

Add two sprigs of rosemary *(Ros-
marinus officinalis)*, one of nature's
best protectors of memory and
invigorators of hair.

Add a handful of sage *(Salvia
officianalis)* leaves if you have dark
hair, or a handful of daisies *(Bellis
perennis)* if you are fair.

Add to a jug or cafetière and pour a
pint of boiling water over. Allow to
steep until cool.

Strain and add five drops of essential oil. Rosemary or peppermint
(Mentha x piperita) will add to
the stimulating nature, chamomile
(Chamaemelum nobile) will make it
soothing and relaxing.

Pour a cupful over the scalp and
massage in, each time before washing and your hair will thank you!

Keeps for a couple of weeks
if chilled.

So many elements of the wild
swan story tell of the reasons why
nettles should be valued. After all,
transformational enchantment
can take unexpected forms and
maybe nettles are just what you
need in a simple **tisane**, infused
for three minutes in freshly boiled
water and drunk to bring life back
to your tired body as you drift into
daydreams of taking swan form!

Or maybe you'd like to try a simple
recipe, using the nettles externally?
One popular in Elizabeth Blackwell's day is a recipe that promised a
lustrous head of youthful hair, one
said to restore hair growth, a scalp
nourishing, invigorating hair rinse.

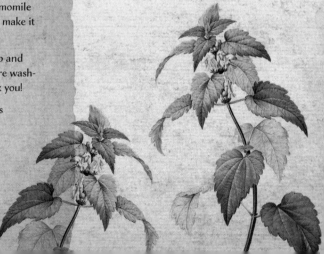

As the story ends, we return to Elizabeth. We hear that the **Witchcraft Act** has finally been revoked. She has successfully had her *Curious Herbal* validated by the Royal College of Physicians and has secured enough income to have her beloved, roguish husband released from prison.

But as we watch and listen he finds himself a new post as 'agricultural advisor' to the King of Sweden – we hear her sigh as she listens to him unveil this latest plan – and she prepares once she has finished her herbal to travel out and join him. Whereupon Alexander finds himself caught up in a Jacobite-influenced plot to fiddle and tweak somewhat the running order for the claim on the Swedish throne and is promptly executed, the harshest cut of all!

She returns home with her child, tears fall as she makes her way back to Chelsea along the banks of the Thames, the early evening crescent moon reflected in dark swirling waters.

It is St Luke's night, the 18th of October. The Syrian doctor we met in Roman times has now become the patron saint of artists and doctors. As Elizabeth arrives home her hands brush through the lavender and she picks the very last of the year's purple spike-flowers and puts them into a cup, pouring on steaming water and allowing it to steep. Three long minutes pass...

She bends over the soft blue-hued infusion and inhales, murmuring words said to help her dream of her lost true love on this night.

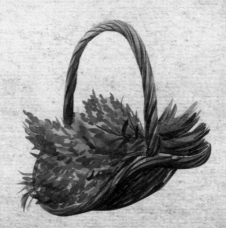

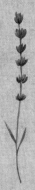

ELIZABETH BLACKWELL'S LAVENDER CHARM TO SEE YOUR TRUE LOVE IN A DREAM

(Helps you see true loves you have yet to meet, just as well, or so the theory goes!)

On the 18th of October, St Luke's day, before going to bed.

Take five stalks of lavender *(Lavandula angustifolia)*, or a teaspoon of dried flowers and steep in a mugful of freshly boiled water for three minutes.

Take a moment to inhale the beautiful, sleep-inducing aroma, allow the steam to gently caress your face. It will help soothe the skin, and a dab of the tea used before bed acts as a wonderful home-made skin toner.

As you start to sip the brew recite the words:

St Luke, St Luke,
Be kind to me
And in my dreams,
Let me my true love see.

I advise a small handsewn pillow – a folded over hanky, stitched round the edge makes a quick pillow - filled with a handful or two of the dried herb to add to this bedtime ritual.

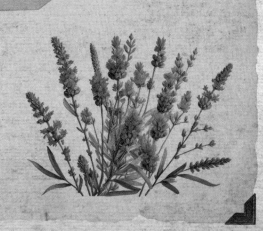

We watch as Elizabeth sips her tea and sings to her child, and we wonder if she will see Alexander in her dreams. Before we slip away, we hope at least that she gets a good night's rest soothed by the soporific lavender and wakes with renewed vigour to keep sharing her pictures of plants.

We then lose track of the curious but wonderful Elizabeth, though we know she is buried just along the road from her beloved Chelsea Physic Garden, at Chelsea Old Parish church. A plaque to her now sits on the church wall alongside one to St Luke – a fitting resting place – and we take our own brew and sip and wonder where we will go next.

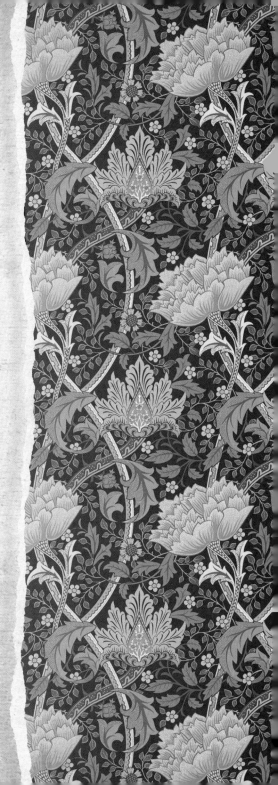

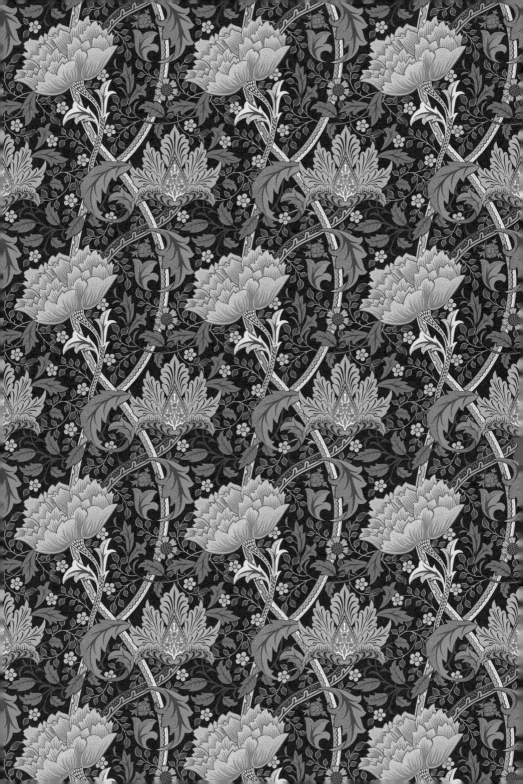

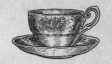

BORDER BALLADS
AND BIRCH

1800

We spiral onwards, but something has changed. There are subtle altera-
tions in the quality of the light, as if the sunrise that greeted us in the last
century and expanded over our time there, the 'enlightenment', has caused
everyone to decide to move faster, do more.

We need to take time to slow down, to contemplate before we continue onwards into time. Hearts pounding as
the speeding spiral threatens to become a vortex, we dig
our heels downwards, towards the earth and anchor in. We
have stopped.

There are beings moving. The moment has come to
listen again and see what is happening in this place.
We are on the edge of a birch wood, and behind us is
a meadow, flooded in patches with ponds almost becoming lochs thanks to recent rains.
Cotton grass (*Eriophorum angustifolium*)
grows around the boggy edges, its white tufted
tops dancing ghost-like in the gloaming.

A child stands with a gathered bundle of the stems in a basket by his feet. He is patiently stripping the green exterior from each stem, revealing the candle-wick centre, and passing them to his mother who carefully places the foamy pith into the basket.

They will become the centre of a candle like the one she carries in a lamp, lighting their way home as early evening takes hold. If there is any to spare it will be saved to dress grazed knees, staunching blood before healing St John's wort (*Hypericum perforatum*) and plantain (*Plantago sp.*) leaf are used as a poultice to speed the skin's recovery.

A stone we recognise from the boundary of the **Pictish** village on one of our earlier journeys, reveals that we are near a place familiar from another of our other stops, but the village has changed once more. New houses have grown up and a group of children now dance around the stone singing:

'Ollie peep, Ollie Peep, here's his heid but whar's his feet?'

It seems that the boundary stone has now gained the moniker 'the De'ils Heid'. He has been buried here a long time, watching the changes take place around him. His home here is still marked by a hawthorn tree clad with berries.

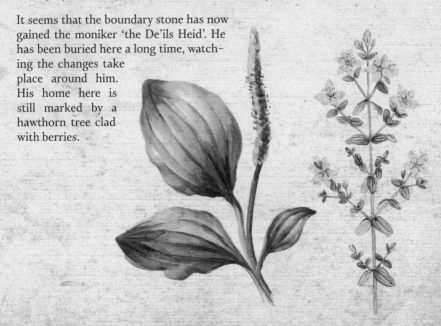

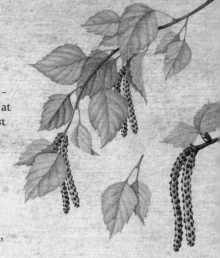

There is an air, an atmosphere, an indication of liminality. We sense that our journey may be ending at least for the time being, but there is another almost otherworldly quality here too.

Our eyes are caught by another group of chanting children, this time carrying a jack o'lantern, a gruesome leering grin, a smell of burning neep and tallow... We have arrived here at **Samhain**, a liminal time indeed, a time to die back to allow for renewal - and behind us is the first plant of renewal, the silver birch (*Betula pendula*).

Birch trees have started to appear between the willows (*Salix sp.*) that once bordered this small loch, a mere dew pond really, but one that like any other edge-dwelling entity appears and disappears according to the surrounding conditions. The trees have pushed up through the moss, gathering as a community, a *corps de ballet*. They invite us to pause.

We dare not move, we sense the trees might be about to pick up their roots and travel down to the water's edge to drink and dance. As we watch I will whisper to you the story of the gifts that trees give, not just the gentle salicylate-raising properties gifted by the willow's bark, or the resinous, cleansing notes from the shallow-rooted pine, but of the jewels that may lie beneath their gnarled old roots and of the fate of one who did not heed a storyteller's warning.

Other stories – of dancing **birch-maidens** – were first gathered, they say, on the Norse trade winds. Whether the kidney-cleansing sweep of birch existed in Scotland before our exchange of stories and cultures with the Scandinavian peoples is almost impossible to tell. Some believe birch may have always been here, some say she came from other lands. But we are an island nation, we have always travelled, exchanging seeds and stories – seas are not barriers but saline, twisted, silver tidal paths.

We know this age is different, this is a time when the world of the other – the dead, the fae, the unfamiliar – and the world of the living have drawn close. The veil is thin and as I have whispered to you the stories of dancing connected to the trees, the children have gathered close. They hear my whisper, we are visible to them in their lantern-light and they gather close, hoping for a tale.

I tell the story told by Duncan Williamson, a traveller's tale of a birch besom seller who created one vast broom for a witch – a big woman who had struggled to find a substantial enough vehicle upon which to fly to reach the witches' Hallowe'en ball. On finally reaching the gathering for the first time, she overhead her sisters laughing that she couldn't get a broom to lift her. So before joining them for the celebrations, she crept around to where they had parked their own brooms and threw them into the branches of the birch canopy, sniggering as they failed to find them at the end of the dance and had to walk wearily home.

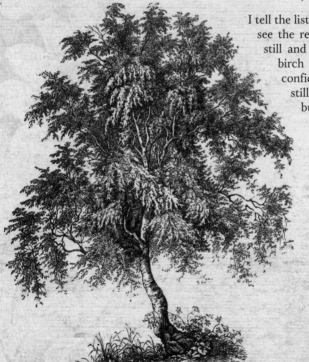

I tell the listening children they can see the remnants of the brooms still and they disperse into the birch trees to find them. I confide to you that they are still there in our own day, but that they are now cunningly disguised as contorted fungal growths (still referred to as 'witches' broom disease'), as the witches have now learnt to disguise their presence with science!

So here we are, gathered in this birch glade where the witches once danced, sensing this may be our last journey, at least for a time.

As we contemplate the world around us, trying to hold on to the memories of the things we have seen, we catch sight of a woman. She has clearly travelled far to reach this magical place. I must look back and tell her tale, because this is a tale that needs to be told, for this is the old wife who lives by Usher's well.

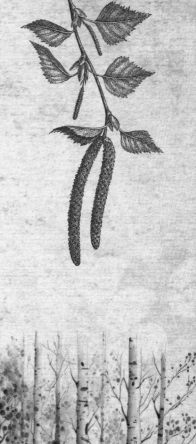

She stands by the trunk of a silver-clad birch watching her child dance. She is clearly glad to see the child happy, but there is deep grief in her eyes, a loss. She is missing the girl's older siblings and she has travelled to this place from her own borderland home, in the hope of tracking down the whereabouts of one of her missing sons. Three have gone before, two she knew had died, but the loss of the third she has just discovered, and the girl does not yet know.

One had been the woman's own flesh and blood, one her cherished stepchild, and one she'd adopted and cared for along the way, when his own mother had been lost in childbirth. But each she loved as much as any mother could love a child.

One had been taken by a fever, one had lost his life in a battle, one it turned out had not been able to meet this life any more... but each had gone and she missed them now more than anything.

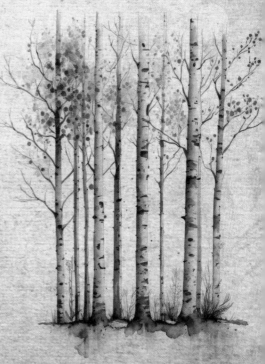

As she stands and watches the child dance, she tap, tap, taps at a silver birch trunk, adding a spile in the hope to draw just a drop of sap out of season, a drop holding the promise of renewal to a heavy heart. For this is the season of **Samhain**, a liminal time where our world is drawn into a different space.

As she tap, tap, taps, one drop falls from the trunk and she wishes:

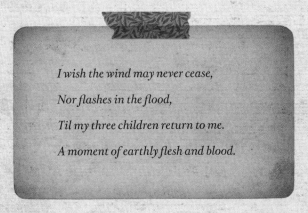

> *I wish the wind may never cease,*
>
> *Nor flashes in the flood,*
>
> *Til my three children return to me.*
>
> *A moment of earthly flesh and blood.*

As she looks from the drop of birch sap outward into the gloaming she sees three figures move as if rising up from the moss itself.

Her three lost bairns.

For they are always her bairns however grown.

Each brow is circled by a coronet of birch, said to protect the dead from the living. Like no other **revenant** they only come to hug their mother and to tell her they are there to watch over her and the youngest child. They do not have a final task. They have not come to tell her to end her grief, as grief does not end it just transforms. They do not stay long, for there was little else to tell. They must go, but new life will follow in their path.

A Birch Tree's Gift for Renewal

Spring birch leaves are traditionally used as a cleansing, refreshing tea. Lightly tannin in flavour, it is said to benefit the kidneys and urinary system, is anti-inflammatory, high in vitamin C, and can assist the body to renew itself, ready for a fresh start. Many people find the taste a little like a fresh green tea and it goes well with a little mint or a slice of lemon added.

BIRCH TREE TEA

On a full moon...

Gather about eight tiny twig tips of birch (small enough to be able to move around in a teacup) and one slightly larger twig.

Gently wash with fresh cold running water.

Bind the small twigs firmly to the bottom of your larger twig. I like to use a nettle string for this, but you may like to try making your own small length of simple plant cordage. This can be done by choosing a flexible plant fibre and either plaiting or twisting.

You now have a small birch whisk with which to stir your tea.

Gather either 27 tiny, fresh green birch leaves on a full moon, when they open in the spring; or dry and save a small amount for use throughout the year. (If leaves are beyond the first bud then use more sparingly, as few as nine may be enough).

Place the leaves directly into your cup, add fresh boiling water, sit and whisk gently with your birch twigs for at least three minutes.

Sip and enjoy, maybe think about renewal...

CAUTION: Birch tree tea can be taken several times a day, but if you are going to drink three cups or more every day, or intend to use it to treat a major health condition, then please consult a qualified medical herbalist first.

She watches as the thread-like **mycelia** winds around their feet, the moss pools around their ankles and they are gone. She gathers up her spile and heals the wound in the tree, then calls to her daughter and walks away. Tomorrow she will tell her daughter all and they will journey back to the borderland cottage by the well. The daughter will tell her mother's story, worked into the lyrics of a song, to a man she works for in Edinburgh, a writer collecting ballads. He will share it in a book and people will love the sadness, and be reassured by the familiar tale of loss. But we have seen it and felt the mother's sense that death is part of life and that everything returns to the soil.

PINE AND BIRCH ROOM MIST

I can't promise that this mist will protect you from the living, unfortunately! However, it will bring some of the cleansing, renewing and revitalising benefits of these two fast-growing trees into your home.

When I'm out and about at workshops and performances I use a room aromatizer to add essential oils and plant essences to a room, to gently bring something of the plants I am telling stories about to the space. In these situations, clearly a naked flame from a candle, or popping a bowl of infused water onto a radiator or by a fire, is impractical. However, for home use a simple ceramic 'oil vaporiser' with a candle is ideal. Suggestions that only oils can be used are simplistic, as although water-based mixtures do evaporate more quickly, they are still a simple sustainable way to use locally foraged or homegrown ingredients to infuse the air. Most herbal teas can be used as a base water, so it's fun to experiment with scents. Alternatively, put your mixture into a glass or ceramic bowl or ramekin and place it on top of a radiator or by a fire to slowly evaporate.

Take a large handful of fresh (or dried) green, spring-harvested birch leaves and place them in a cafetiere (or a warm cup).

Add 140ml (¼ pint) boiling water.

Allow to infuse for seven minutes.

Strain.

Add five to eight drops of Scots pine (*Pinus silvestris*) essential oil. It is worth seeking out a good quality specific Scots pine oil as the aroma is more subtle and sophisticated.

If Scots pine essential oil is not available a strong decoction of fresh (unsprayed) pine needles can be used. Just simmer a few twigs and a handful of needles in water for around ten minutes and strain. The aroma is not as intense, however, if you prefer a real Christmas tree, then this is a lovely way to use it at the end of its time. Alternatively, a few twigs can easily be found in the wild. Any pine species can be used, but make sure you can safely identify it, as yew (*Taxus baccata*) looks pine-like and most parts are extremely toxic!

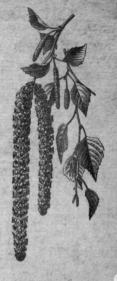

Optional: 10ml (⅓fl oz) single malt whisky can be added. Not only does it add a beautiful peaty aroma, it will also help preserve the liquid so it will keep for several weeks.

Keep in a bottle that can safely be shaken well before a little is poured into the bowl (or the bottle of your aromatiser).

The birch is associated with the Scottish practice of **saining**, which uses smoke to cleanse a space. Pine has benefits for the respiratory system and is associated with promoting a sense of health and wellbeing. It is also invigorating so maybe best not used at bedtime!

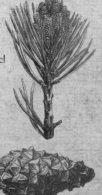

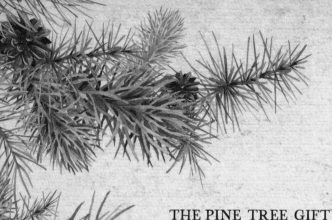

THE PINE TREE GIFT

Birch is a pioneer species, reclaiming land scarred by humans and allowing a second tree, pine, to seed and continue the process. I'd like to take a moment and share a story with you of that second tree...

I was once caught late at night, in a violent storm. As I got to the bridge leading to my house, I was greeted by the sight of fifteen mature pine trees torn down by the wind, blocking my path, with the gale still howling through the remaining wood. I had to get home so, terrified and calling out loud to the trees not to fall on me, I climbed over the immense trunks and through dense branches, homeward.

The next morning the storm was spent, so I ventured out and gathered pine-cones from the fallen trees. Reaching out to caress the bark of the last fallen giant, I murmured thanks to them for letting me get home safely the night before. Taking the cones, I added them to a burgeoning basket of collected woodland herbal treasures – twists of birch bark paper, juniper and rowan berries – things that would find their way into stories, like the one I'm about to tell you now.

We'll need to traverse old, forgotten pathways, stepping round ivy clad trunks that harbour small birds trembling from the cold north wind, past the green lichen-furred oak, until we find ourselves outside a cottage in a clearing at the heart of the wood.

In the cottage live a family, poor in gold but rich in love.

There is a pot of stew simmering on the fire and the scent of pine resin fills the air. The food might be poor, the night bitterly cold, and there may be the sound of a distant storm brewing, but it's a well-loved home and the family are happy.

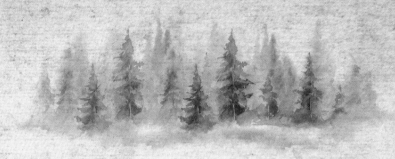

We watch through the veil of trees and time as the night closes in and snow starts to fall. There is only the sound of the wind, lifting and blowing the feather-like drifting of snow. Then softly, the sense of presence, footsteps walking through the snow, a gentle tap at the larchwood door.

An old woman stands outside, flakes flurry around her. The family cannot believe this ancient figure has travelled on this ominous night. They usher her in, welcome her to share their food and their fire, and to join them as they tell stories. It is longest night, and outside snow clouds have smothered the stars. The moon is enveloped in a diaphanous chiffon of ice. They make her a bed for the night.

Morning is chill, but the crystal-tinted sun filters through and the family rise with the bright winter light. Expecting to share their meagre breakfast with their strange visitor, the children make their way downstairs to find her gone. They rush to the door.

She isn't in sight, not even a footprint in the snow shows where she has been.

But outside the door the pine tree at the heart of the forest now stands covered in stars, twinkling and magical. And on the once bare table in the cottage there now sits a hearty meal.

From that day on, so the trees tell me, on longest night the family receive a meal and a tree covered in stars as a gift for helping a poor old woman with the last they had to share.

We slip away. We are about to return to our own hearths, protected by the things gathered from the woods. We light a fire to stop the **Cailleach** grasping at our bones, we **coorie** in, we rest as winter comes and await the shift back into the light.

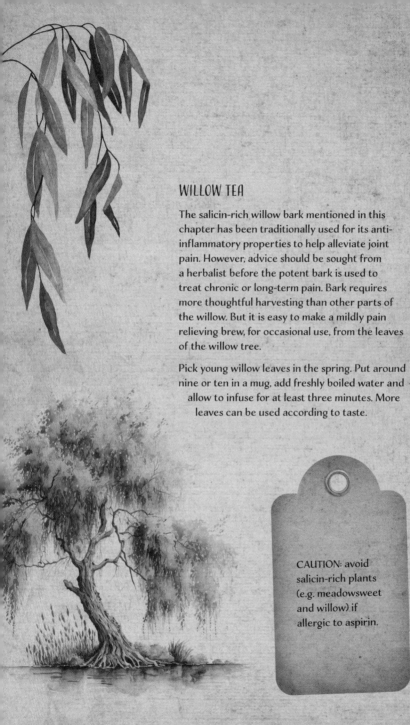

WILLOW TEA

The salicin-rich willow bark mentioned in this chapter has been traditionally used for its anti-inflammatory properties to help alleviate joint pain. However, advice should be sought from a herbalist before the potent bark is used to treat chronic or long-term pain. Bark requires more thoughtful harvesting than other parts of the willow. But it is easy to make a mildly pain relieving brew, for occasional use, from the leaves of the willow tree.

Pick young willow leaves in the spring. Put around nine or ten in a mug, add freshly boiled water and allow to infuse for at least three minutes. More leaves can be used according to taste.

CAUTION: avoid salicin-rich plants (e.g. meadowsweet and willow) if allergic to aspirin.

As we prepare to leave this time with its overwhelming sense of loss, and a rapidly encroaching period of change of the horizon, we realise our journey is coming to an end.

The birch and then the pine stretch out their roots in an attempt to re-wild land cleared for sheep, where the ancient oaks have been harvested for their tannins and also to provide the ships needed to explore new lands and create trade routes. We know that the work of the trees has barely even begun, because there is more change coming, and they will need to remember their role in reclaiming the environment because they will soon be needed more than ever.

Maybe we can help them if we grasp a few birch twigs, verdant with leaves, as the time spiral beckons us again and we take a deep breath and settle, ready for our last journey.

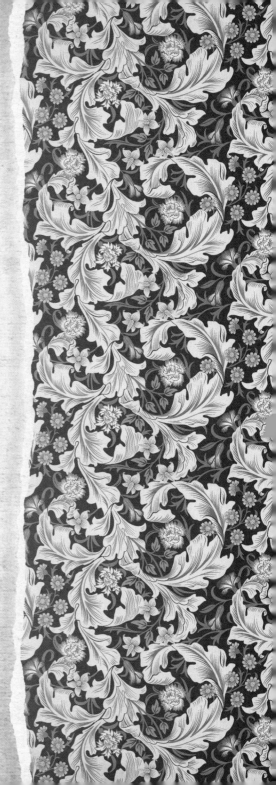

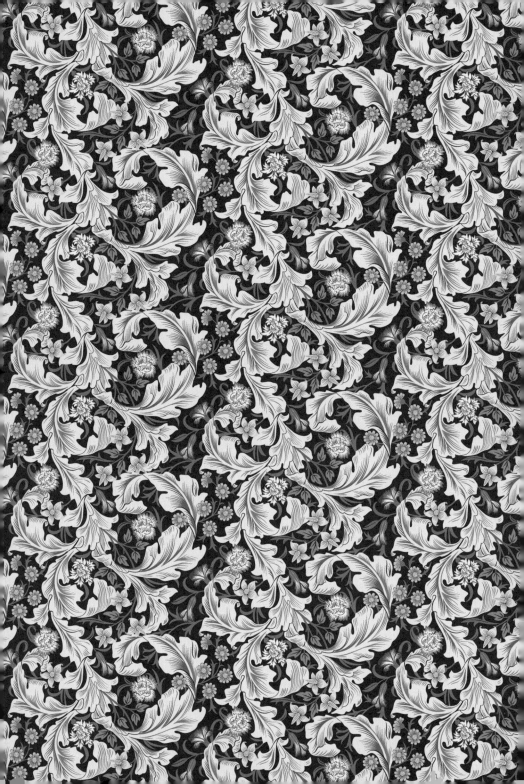

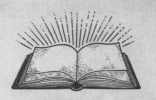

RETURNING

Returning hame, from whence you came,

Count back up and down again.

Eenerie, twaaerie, tuckery seven,

Halipa, crackapa, tenapa 'leven,

Pin pan musky dan,

Eidlum tweetlum twenty wan.

You are now IN.

Traditional children's rhyme

Take another breath, slowly look around you, we have returned to our own time it would seem, and for now our time travelling must pause. Two hundred years hovers in front of us, appealing, encouraging, inviting us to step into its path. But we sense minds intent on mastering money, seeking to licence and hold the ancient cures we have come to accept as gifts on our journey, and we know there are huge changes about to come. We sense a world that changes faster than at any time we have yet experienced, so we suspect we had better pause and steel ourselves for a faster journey next time we meet. We are about to face an industrial era, and we had best get ready for a rapid input of information.

MINT TEA

There are oral records of wild mint being used in an infusion to clear the head and aid the digestion from the Isle of Tiree, off Scotland's west coast, in the early 19th century. The same uses are associated with mint tea around the world. In some traditions it is said to be effective at getting rid of what is no longer useful and creating a sense of wonder, inspiration, and newness – so it might be the perfect drink to sip on our return!

Take a teaspoon of dried mint or nine fresh leaves.

Steep in a mug of freshly boiled water for three minutes.

Strain and sip with a piece of freshly baked Scots gingerbread perhaps…?

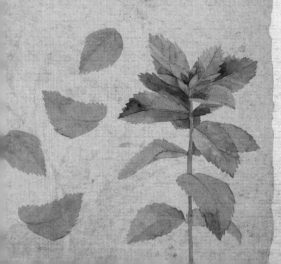

We sense that the fear of witches has now almost entirely vanished. **Revenants,** unearthly beings and vampiric **Striga**, once accepted or held at bay just by healing plants and turnip lanterns, are being trapped in fairy tales for children by enlightenment and encroaching industrial enterprises.

But we still hear whispers from the church that there is trouble to be found in the culture of men and women studying botany together. **Mary Wollstonecraft** has been reviled by men of power for her *Vindication of the Rights of Women*, and women seem to be being forced to take a step backwards, rather than one forwards in time. We wonder where those hidden recipes will go, and we want to find them and hold them before they vanish.

But for now, we must stop and ground ourselves, consolidate and test the recipes we have found. And the best way to ground yourself? Well of course I want to return to the place where this all began, in my gran's kitchen, feet on the cold floor, warming ginger and iron-rich treacle scenting the air. Maybe a cup of digestion-easing peppermint tea to clear the head…

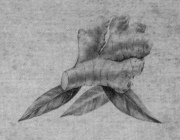

As the Scots gingerbread recipe given here is one collected by McNeill, there are no precise instructions for the modern cook, but my gran's annotations in the margin of my copy of the book confirm my memories of her baking it, and the smell transports me back to childhood.

By the way, if you're after a modern translation, the amounts are as follows: 340g (12oz) flour, 115g (4oz) oatmeal, 225g (8oz) butter, 30g (1oz) green ginger, 115g (4oz) lemon peel, 340g (12oz) treacle and 70ml (5fl oz) cream. The original recipe doesn't specify an oven temperature, but 180ºC (355ºF) should be about right. Ten minutes before the end of the cooking time, check with a clean knife/skewer to see if the gingerbread is cooked through (the knife should come out cleanly). If necessary cover the gingerbread with foil if it starts to look too brown on the top.

When I make the cake, I adapt it to suit the ingredients available, using a teaspoon of dried ginger and the same weight as suggested of crystallised ginger, instead of green, and finely grating the lemon. I also often substitute half the treacle for honey as it has a lighter flavour. Although

SCOTS GINGERBREAD

A traditional recipe (with original instructions) from Florence Marian McNeill's *The Scots Kitchen*:

Flour, oatmeal, butter, green ginger, lemon peel, treacle, cream.

Beat eight ounces of butter to a cream. Mix with it twelve ounces of flour, four ounces of oatmeal, and half a gill of cream.

Stir in twelve ounces of treacle, one ounce of green ginger, and four ounces of lemon peel cut into fine shreds.

Work the whole into a light dough.

Put in a well-greased tin and bake for forty-five minutes.

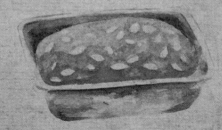

GINGER – THE SPICE OF LIFE

'And I had but one penny in the world, thou should'st have it to buy gingerbread.'

from *Love's Labour's Lost* by William Shakespeare

Gingerbread has changed form in almost every era that we have travelled through...

Merchants have sprinkled a little powdered ginger into their pockets and purses to attract wealth, and the wealthy folk they sold it to have encased chunks of the fresh root in bread to end banquets, promising their guests it would aid their digestion. Witches have built appetising houses from it, in the hope children wouldn't undo their hard work, and Good Queen Bess has had her cooks construct sweet ginger facsimiles of her visiting guests to curry favour.

For the duration of our travels, the nausea-relieving properties of ginger and its abilities to add warmth to dishes – written about in the first century in *De Materia Medica* by Pedanius Dioscorides, Greek medical botanist and physician who served in the Roman army – has been commonly accepted. Now research is also going on to give scientific authority to other time-tested ancient uses. We are turning to ginger for its anti-inflammatory properties, its ability to alleviate joint pain.

Maybe, as Confucius suggested in 479BC, we should eat it at every meal.

the traditional version calls for 4oz of lemon, I find this quite a lot. The grated zest of one large lemon should be sufficient, but do experiment and adapt to suit.

In the footnotes of her book Mc-Neill writes of silver charms being put in cakes for Hallowe'en, charms that foretold a future for someone who found them in their slice. You could add a ring, to suggest a union or marriage, a coin for wealth, a wish-bone for 'the heart's desire', or horseshoe for good luck, or maybe you could create charms with associated meanings unique to you, and embed them in a folkloric cake all of your own.

Ginger is relatively high in vitamin B6 and magnesium, so my suggestion that this is grounding is supported by the mood-improving effect of these nutrients. Oats in herbal medicine are attributed with qualities that soothe the nerves and create calm within the body, and the treacle is rich in iron, so this gingerbread may be the perfect food to restore us after a journey.

So as you sip your tea and wait for the cake to cool a little, I will bid you goodbye, until we gather again, to step into the spiral and discover a new era and more stories from the back of the apothecary's cabinet!

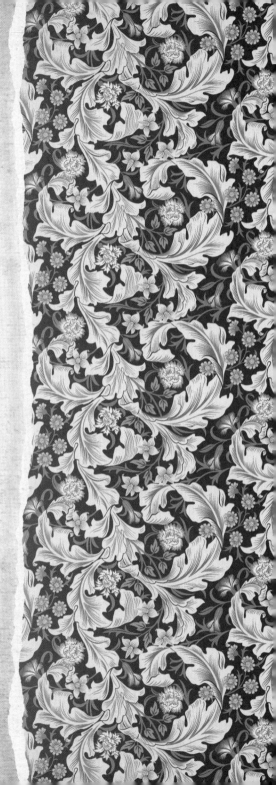

GLOSSARY

Bannock: An unleavened, flat, unsweetened cake traditionally made in Scotland of oats and occasionally of barley.

Bennu: The story of the Bennu – a phoenix-like bird of Eyptian mythology – can be found in a number of texts (one of the earliest is by Greek scholar Herodotus in the fifth century BC), and is also referred to in scientific research. See A.S. Haffor and A. Rajabian *et al* in the bibliography.

Birch-maidens: Folkloric figures who inhabit and embody the spirit of birch trees. The story goes that they loved to dance and might reward those who danced with them.

Birls (Scots dialect): Turns around or spins on the spot.

Cailleach: Known as the Queen of Winter or The Veiled One, the Cailleach was one of the great Celtic ancestors, and goddess of the cold and the winds. In legend, she controlled the length and harshness of winter.

Caointeach: A strange supernatural figure who washes the linen of those who will die, in a stream, usually by their home. In some stories, she is encountered on a journey. She often keens or cries (like the Irish banshee) but although she can be malicious if you interrupt her task, she does not seek to do any harm. She realises her tidings can be hard to hear!

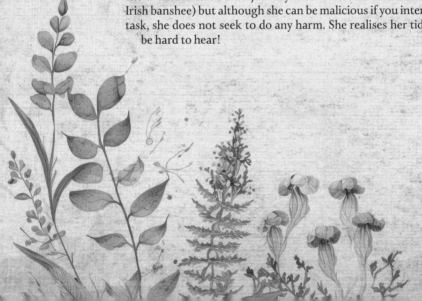

Carse (Scots dialect): a fertile, lowland area, usually boggy and by a river.

Coorie (Scot's dialect): To stoop, cringe or crouch for protection and shelter, or to nestle for comfort.

Cu Chulainn: A warrior hero most closely associated with the Irish Ulster Cycles, but who also appears in Scottish and Manx folklore.

Cystoliths: Microscopic rods of calcium carbonate, which can be absorbed by the body and may interfere with kidney function.

Eleanor of Aquitaine (1122-1204): Heiress, first married to Louis VII of France and later married to Henry II of England. Understood to have been well read and learned in healing traditions herself (see Elisabeth Brooke in the bibliography). She was also the founder of healing orders, a tradition that her female descendants continued.

Eòlas (Scots dialect): A traditional spell, charm or incantation, usually containing magical knowledge.

Fairy howe: A mound or hill associated with fairies.

Frith (Scots dialect): without an accent this is something small, a small charm. Alternatively 'frìth' (with an accent over the i) is an augury or divination, potentially in a rhyme.

Gregorian calendar: Introduced by Pope Gregory the XIII to replace the Julian calendar in 1562, it was designed to balance the leap year making the calendar follow the solar year more closely.

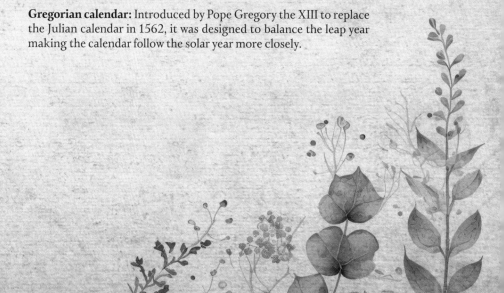

Hildegard of Bingen: A twelfth-century German polymath, later sanctified, who collected and aligned classical and folk-medicine belief and who wrote and theorised extensively on medicine, developing ideas that contributed significantly to the treatment of disease at the time.

Hogmanay (Scot's dialect): The last day of the year, otherwise known as New Year's Eve.

Isobella MacDuff's court: The first copy of a Syrian manuscript containing the three hundred tales that we associate with *A Thousand and One Arabian Nights*, which contains the tale of **Tawaddud** referenced in my story of Isobella, is recorded as being in the collection of the Bibliothèque Nationale de France in around 1350. It was a time when the silk and spice roads still brought merchants with tales to share to wealthy families. The French barons had risen to power in the UK and the Scottish Royal Burghs held profitable rights to trade spices. This period seems to have inspired many of the later French and Italian literary fairy tales we often find familiar in modern Western cultures. The allusion to Petrosinella, Rapunzel and Sleeping Beauty, explored through historical female healers of the period in the 'Spices, Fairytales and Plague' chapter, is influenced by these factors. **Isobella MacDuff**, Countess of Fife, was a real person, her lineage and personal circumstances are based on facts, but the details of her story in this book are merely constructed from memories of our time travelling adventures!

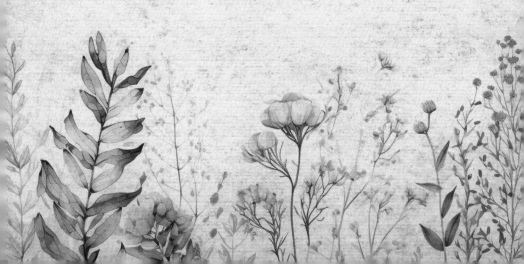

Inulins: Naturally occurring polysaccharides produced by plants, which act as a prebiotic and improve digestive health, and may boost the immune system.

Janus: The ancient Roman god with two faces, one looking forward, one back. Janus is associated with gateways, transitions, doorways and new beginnings.

Kirk (Scots and northern English dialect): The church, more specifically used in Scotland on occasion to refer to the Church of Scotland.

Mary Wollstonecraft (1759–1797): English writer, philosopher and advocate of women's rights.

The Morrigan: A figure from Irish mythology, whose name translates as 'phantom queen'. Often depicted as a triple goddess, she is associated with not only war and fate but also with guardianship of the land or the earth. She is said to be capable of transformation. She appears in both the Ulster Cycles, on which my interpretation is loosely based, and the Mythological Cycles.

Mycelia (plural of mycelium): The mass of branched, tubular filaments (hyphae) of fungi. Understood to act as a communication network supporting the fruiting bodies, the plants and soil they grow in community with.

Oxymel: a liquid – often a blend of water, honey and vinegar – infused with herbs and reduced to a syrup.

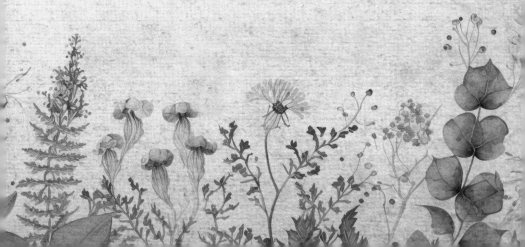

Philosopher's stone: A legendary alchemical item, capable of turning base metals into gold, sometimes also said to be capable of gifting eternal life.

Picts/Pictish: The name Pict (meaning painted people) was the term given to the tribes of northern Scotland, probably by the Romans. At the time of writing, a lot of our beliefs about the Pictish tribes is speculation, with clues hidden in the fragments of stories that may date back to Late Antiquity, and the symbols carved into the beautiful stones we associate with their culture.

Revenant: From the old French word for 'returning', revenants occur throughout folklore, often as animated corpses (although the term also used to refer to ghosts) to haunt the living. In Scottish lore the tradition is that they are often benign and have returned to either complete an unfinished task or to tell a loved one that the time for intense grief has passed. Traditionally this was after a year and a day.

Rosemary Gladstar: American herbalist and author, founder of United Plant Savers.

Saining (Scots dialect): traditional Scottish practice of cleansing using a smouldering smoke.

Salicylates: Plant chemicals that have a protective and preserving benefit within plant cells. Traditionally these plants have been used by herbalists as anti-inflammatories and for pain relief. In modern times we have isolated and replicated these to create a group of salicylate drugs such as aspirin (salicylic acid). This derivative of salicylate can be found in plants like willow trees and myrtle. It is used in 'over the counter' and prescription medicines for its analgesic, anti-inflammatory and antipyretic (temperature lowering) properties.

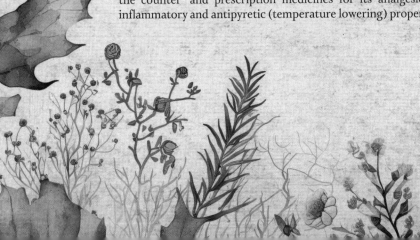

Samhain: Perhaps better known now as Hallowe'en, this festival has ancient Celtic roots, originating in Ireland and in Scotland. It marked the Celtic new year, the time of year when the veil is thinnest between worlds and it is easiest to contact the otherworld. Traditionally a fire festival, it is celebrated halfway between the autumn equinox and winter solstice.

Striga (singular, strix): A bird of ill omen, which was said to have been created by metamorphosis in classical mythology. In his *Fasti*, Ovid described the strix as a 'large-headed bird with transfixed eyes, rapacious beak, greyish white wings and hooked claws...'. Striga were said to feed on the flesh and blood of people, and in particular that of children. Later the term was extended to cover witches, the Italian word 'strega' (meaning 'witch') is derived from the term.

Tairsgear (Scots dialect): An implement used for peat cutting.

Tawaddud: 'The Slave Girl of Tawaddud' is a tale from *A Thousand and One Arabian Nights*, in which a slave girl proves herself with her incredible knowledge and saves her master from poverty. She is freed as a reward but elects to stay with him as his companion.

Tisane: A medicinal drink or infusion, usually a herbal tea, made by steeping plant ingredients in boiling water.

Trotula of Salerno: A physician and an instructor at the School of Salerno in Italy in the twelfth century, and one of the most famous physicians of the time. She wrote extensively on medicine, her most famous work being *Passionibus Mulierum Curandorum (The Diseases of Women)*, also known as *Trotula Major*.

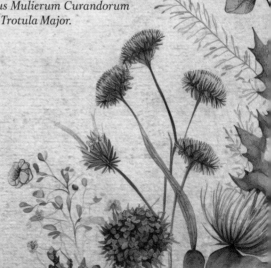

Urisk: A folkloric creature of Scottish mythology, akin to the brownie or broonie, so on occasion it will help with tasks on the land or in the home. However, the Urisk, unlike the broonie, is more commonly found in lonely wild places, often by a waterfall. It is said to be wild and hairy and very protective of its wild natural space.

Well kent (Scots dialect): Well known.

The Wild Hunt: A folkloric legend of a hunt that indicates a forthcoming battle or plague, often lead by a legendary figure. In Scandinavian mythology this was often Odin, in British myths it can also be lead by the fairy queen intent on abducting a human.

The Witchcraft Act: First passed by parliament in 1542, this Act made witchcraft punishable by death. It was swiftly revoked, only to be replaced in 1562. During the reign of James I, who took a keen interest in witchcraft and demonology, a further law was passed, in 1604. The 1562 and 1604 Acts transferred the responsibility for the trial of witches from the Church to the secular courts.

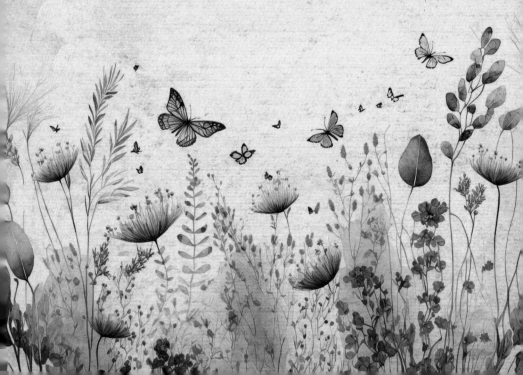

RESOURCES

The register of professional medical herbalists in the UK is curated by the **National Institute of Medical Herbalists.** To contact this organisation or to find a herbalist visit www.nimh.org.uk. The US equivalent is the **American Herbalists Guild,** which can found at: www.americanherbalistsguild.com

Another source of information on herbal plants and their uses is **The Herbal Society of Great Britain.** Its aim is to support the practice of herbal medicine in Britain. They can be found here: www.herbsociety.org.uk

One of my favourite resources for uncovering the memories, stories and traditions of Scotland is Tobar an Dualchais, which is free to access and can be found here: https://www.tobaranddualchais.co.uk. **Tobar an Dualchais/Kist o Riches** is Scotland's online resource dedicated to the presentation and promotion of audio recordings of Scotland's cultural heritage. Its principal content is songs, music, history, poetry, traditions and stories, recorded from the 1930s onwards.

If you've been inspired to read more of **Elizabeth Blackwell's A Curious Herbal,** you can find a digitised version of it on The British Library's website here: https://www.bl.uk/turning-the-pages/?id=635a7cc0-a675-11db-a027-0050c2490048&ctype=book or on the New York Public Library website here: https://digitalcollections.nypl.org/collections/a-curious-herbal-containing-five-hundred-cuts-of-the-most-useful-plants-which-2#/?tab=navigation

Eliza Smith's Compleat Housewife of 1737 can also be found online here: https://www.google.co.uk/books/edition/The_Compleat_Housewife_Or_Accomplish_d_G/XvMHAAAAQAAJ?hl=en&gbpv=1

I'd like to add a special mention here of my storytelling ecologist friend Lisa Schneidau's book *Botanical Folk Tales of Britain and Ireland* (History Press, 2018). Lisa and I share story threads, though her tales focus on environmental issues and mine on how plants connect us. I would like to acknowledge that she and I collaborated on 'Scotia Botanica' for the Scottish International Storytelling Festival 2022, and elements of the Moss Lights chapter draw on the piece I wrote and performed as part of it.

BIBLIOGRAPHY

Beith, Mary, 'Healing Threads', *Traditional Medicines of the Highlands and Islands* (Polygon, 1995)

Blackwell, Elizabeth, *A Curious Herbal: Containing five hundred cuts, of the most useful plants, which are now used in the practice of physick* (London, 1737)

Brooke, Elisabeth, *Women Healers through History* (The Women's Press Ltd., 1993; new edition Aeon Press, 2020)

Cannone, Nicoletta, Dalle Fratte, Michele, Convey, Peter, Worland, M. Roger, Guglielmin, Mauro, 'Ecology of moss banks on Signy Island (maritime Antarctic)', *Botanical Journal of the Linnean Society*, August 2017; 184 (4)

Carmicheal, Alexander, *Carmina Gadelica, Volume 2* (Oliver & Boyd, 1900)

Chaucer, Geoffrey, *The Canterbury Tales* (Penguin Books, 2007)

Coates, Doris E., *Tuppenny Rice and Treacle: Cottage Housekeeping 1900–1920* (Harpsden Press, 1976)

Cottle, Amos Simon, *Icelandic Poetry* (Bristol, 1797)

Dioscorides P., *De Materia Medica: Being an herbal with many other medicinal materials, written in Greek in the first century of the common era, a new indexed version in modern English,* edited by Osbaldeston, T. A., and Wood, R. P. (Johannesburg, 2000)

Haffor, A.S., 'Effect of myrrh (Commiphora molmol) on leukocyte levels before and during healing from gastric ulcer or skin injury', *Journal of Immunotoxicology*, March 2010; 7(1)

Hotaling, Scott, Bartholomaus, Timothy C., Gilbert, Sophie L., 'Rolling stones gather moss: movement and longevity of moss balls on an Alaskan glacier', *Polar Biology Journal* (2020)

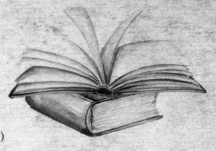

Kirk, Robert, and Lang, Andrew, *The Secret Commonwealth of Elves, Fauns and Fairies* (London, 1893)

Mabinogion, The, translated by Lady Charlotte Guest (Longmans, London, 1877)

MacLean, John, *Balach na h-aimhreit*. This song about the herd boys of Caolas is available from the Tobar an Dualchais/Kiat o Riches archive. MacLean (1787-1848) was bard to the Laird of Coll.

McNeill, F. Marian, *The Scots Kitchen: Its Traditions and Lore, with Old Time Recipes* (Blackie & Son, 1929)

McNeill, F. Marian, *The Silver Bough: A Four Volume Study of the National and Local Festivals of Scotland* (William McLellan, Glasgow 1977)

Moote, A. Lloyd and Dorothy C., *The Great Plague: The Story of London's Most Deadly Year* (The Johns Hopkins University Press, Baltimore, 2006)

Ovid, *Fasti*, translated by Anne and Peter Wiseman (Oxford University Press, 2013)

Pennant, T., *A Tour in Scotland* (London, 1769)

Polson, A., *Our Highland Folklore Heritage* (1926)

Rajabian, A., Sadeghnia, H., Fanoudi, S., Hosseini, A., 'Genus *Boswellia* as a new candidate for neurodegenerative disorders', *Iranian Journal of Basic Medical Sciences*, 2020 Mar; 23(3)

Scott, Walter, *Minstrelsy of the Scottish Border: Consisting of Historical and Romantic Ballads, Collected in the Southern Counties of Scotland; With a Few of Modern Date, Founded Upon Local Tradition. In Two Volumes.* Vol. I (II) (Cadell & Davies, 1802)

Sinclair, Lilia, and Holohan, Clare, *Scotland's Wild Medicine* (Heal Scotland Books, 2020)

Tongue, Ruth L., *Somerset Folklore* (The Folkore Society, 1965)

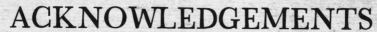

ACKNOWLEDGEMENTS
MY THANKS TO...

My brilliant storytelling mum, Jean Edmiston, and her father, my grandfather, sculptor Richard Ross Robertson RSA for telling me some of the legends that are in the book (principally my retelling of 'The Maidenstone at the Chapel of Garriochmill', an Aberdeenshire legend); and my maternal grandmother Kathleen May Robertson (née Matts) for memories and recipes.

My late mother-in-law Sheena Ritchie for sharing her garden, love of cooking and books, which made me feel like I was comfortably in my own positive, familial time spiral.

Herbalists whom I have encountered and learnt from along the way: Rosemary Gladstar, Elisabeth Brooke and Christopher Hedley for recipes and techniques that have encouraged me to learn from plants, and that I refer to here. And to the Scottish School of Herbal Medicine for starting my formal herbal learning journey.

Libraries, librarians and curators who have found me books and booked me for events that have led to adventures that became stories: the Royal College of Physicians and Surgeons, Glasgow; The Ashmolean Museum, Oxford; The National Library of Scotland; Chelsea Physic Garden; and Aberdeen University Special Collection, amongst many others.

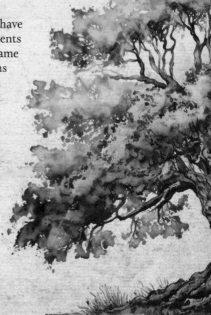

And to many other folk, but a special mention goes to Dr Valentina Bold and DeeDee Chainey (Folklore Thursday) for encouraging me and getting me to write my live storytelling work down, and then reading it and telling me it was worth doing.

ABOUT THE AUTHOR

Once described, by a workshop participant as 'Creating verbal, herbal magic', Amanda Edmiston comes from a long line of storytellers and plant people. She was brought up believing that knowledge of legends, fairy tales, history, art and plants was vital to life. At university she first studied law, imagining a glorious career upholding human rights, before being thwarted by the stressful system. She then studied herbal medicine but elected not to go into clinical practice when she became a mum. Finally, fed up with not knowing what she would do with her life, she invented 'herbal storytelling' and has since developed a professional practice that shares her passion, thanks to the never-failing belief of her mother, artist and storyteller, Jean Edmiston.

Since 2011, Amanda has woven words for Chelsea Physic Garden, taken Scottish folklore and plant use to the National Museum of Rural Life in Scotland and the Ashmolean Museum in Oxford, and shared historical secrets at the Royal College of Physicians and Surgeons, Glasgow. She has also created work for schools and organisations in China, America and Singapore. She also collects stories and memories of plant use from across rural Scotland, to share with her *Kist in Thyme* projects. Much of this heritage wisdom has found its way into *The Time Traveller's Herbal*.

Amanda lives not far from the meadow she talks of in this book, in rural Scotland, with her brilliant, handsome and hugely supportive husband (who did not write this biography, despite being asked), her two beautiful but distracting children and an energetic springer spaniel.

Amanda is an associate member of The National Institute of Medical Herbalists. Discover more about Amanda and Botanica Fabula on her website: www.botanicafabula.co.uk.

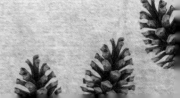

INDEX

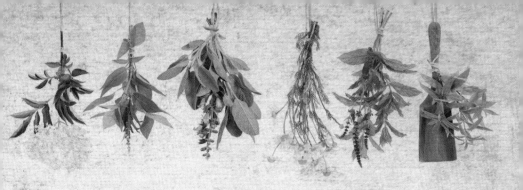

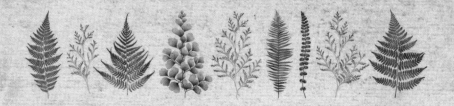

A DAVID AND CHARLES BOOK
© David and Charles, Ltd 2023

David and Charles is an imprint of David and Charles, Ltd, Suite A, Tourism House, Pynes Hill, Exeter, EX2 5WS

Text © Amanda Edmiston 2023
Layout © David and Charles, Ltd 2023

First published in the UK and USA in 2023

Amanda Edmiston has asserted her right to be identified as author of this work in accordance with the Copyright, Designs and Patents Act, 1988.

The author and publisher have made every effort to ensure that all the recipes in the book are accurate and safe, and therefore cannot accept liability for any resulting injury, damage or loss to persons or property, however it may arise.

Names of organisations, people, books and products are provided for the information of readers, with no intention to infringe copyright or trademarks.

A catalogue record for this book is available from the British Library.

ISBN-13: 9781446309919 paperback
ISBN-13: 9781446309735 EPUB
ISBN-13: 9781446310403 PDF

This book has been printed on paper from approved suppliers and made from pulp from sustainable sources.

Printed in China through Asia Pacific Offset for: David and Charles, Ltd, Suite A, Tourism House, Pynes Hill, Exeter, EX2 5WS

10 9 8 7 6 5 4 3 2 1

Publishing Director: Ame Verso
Senior Commissioning Editor: Lizzie Kaye
Managing Editor: Jeni Chown
Copy Editor: Jane Trollope
Head of Design: Anna Wade
Designers: Sam Staddon & Sarah Rowntree
Pre-press Designer: Susan Reansbury
Production Manager: Beverley Richardson

David and Charles publishes high-quality books on a wide range of subjects. For more information visit www.davidandcharles.com.

Follow us on Instagram by searching for @dandcbooks_wellbeing.

Layout of the digital edition of this book may vary depending on reader hardware and display settings.